HIV TESTING

Edited by **Ricardo Sobhie Diaz**

HIV Testing
Edited by Ricardo Sobhie Diaz

Published by InTech
Janeza Trdine 9, 51000 Rijeka, Croatia

Publishing Process Manager Oliver Kurelic

Technical Editor Teodora Smiljanic

Cover Designer InTech Design Team

Additional hard copies can be obtained from orders@intechopen.com

HIV Testing, Edited by Ricardo Sobhie Diaz
p. cm.
ISBN 978-953-307-871-7

For EU product safety concerns:
IN TECH d.o.o., Prolaz Marije Krucifikse Kozulić 3, 51000 Rijeka, Croatia,
info@intechopen.com or visit our website at intechopen.com.

Meet the editor

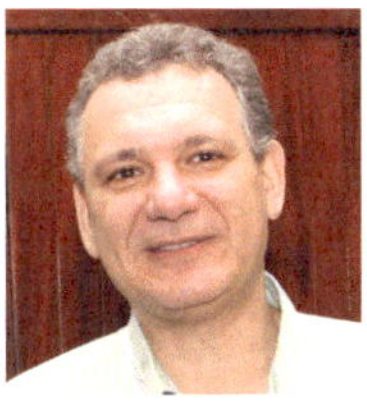

Ricardo Sobhie Diaz is an expert physician with a training in infectious diseases, conducting translational research in HIV/AIDS. He is a professor at the Infectious Diseases Department of Paulista School of Medicine at the Federal University of Sao Paulo, Brazil, and has over 100 articles published in peer-reviewed scientific journals. He is also a member of the "Brazilian Consensus Guidelines for Antiretrovirals for Adults and Adolescents of the Brazilian Ministry of Health", and acts as a consultant in the area of Laboratory of STD/AIDS and Viral Hepatitis Department of the Brazilian Ministry of Health. Dr Diaz is an elected governing council member of the International AIDS Society, representing Latin America and the Carribean.

Contents

Preface

As of 2010, an estimated 34 million individuals (ranging from 31,6 to 35,2 million) are living with HIV according to UNAIDS. There were also 2,7 million new HIV infections in the last year (2,4 to 2,9 million) and 1,8 million (1,6 to 1,9 million) individuals died during last year. It is also estimated that as many as 97% of infections occur in countries of low and median income. Especially vulnerable are women and children in developing countries. Almost 48% of new infections occurred among women and 42% among young people from 15 to 24 years of age.

HIV testing is entering a new era with important considerations for maintaining health and reducing the spreading of the virus. HIV-infected individuals not aware of the infection are not able to take advantage of the therapies that can keep them healthy and extend their lives, nor do they have the knowledge to protect their offspring, and sex or drug-use partners from becoming infected. Knowing whether one is positive or negative for HIV confers great benefits in health decision-making.

The biomedical interventions towards the decrease of HIV-1 transmission have greatly improved in the recent years. One of the factors for decreasing new HIV infections is more effective antiretroviral therapy. In developing world, the effective treatment of HIV infected pregnant women has rendered achievable the virtual elimination of pediatric HIV disease. It has also been demonstrated that HIV treatment of HIV-1 infected individuals can decrease the HIV transmission among discordant couples,[1] meaning that widespread antiretroviral treatment can greatly decrease the HIV-1 transmission in the world,[2] thus configuring the so called "test and treat era". This rationale has become one of the pillars of earlier initiation of antiretroviral therapy in more recent guidelines in Europe and United States, such as the European AIDS Guidelines, the IAS-USA guidelines and the DHHS guidelines. In the absence of an effective HIV vaccine and the lack of adherence to the use of condoms, biomedical interventions, such as male circumcision, have also been advocated as a possible tool for decreasing HIV incidence.[3] Nonetheless, being aware of HIV-1 status is the central pillar of HIV prevention and interruption of HIV-1 transmission chains.

In this book, some original work is presented adding important information on epidemiology of HIV in developing countries *vis a vis* the diagnosis of HIV infection.

Also presented are reviews on the state-of-the-art diagnosis of HIV infection, as well as modern tools that can be used currently and in the future.

Ricardo Sobhie Diaz
Infectious Diseases Division of the Paulista School of Medicine
at the Federal University of Sao Paulo,
Brazil

References

[1] Cambiano V, Rodger AJ, Phillips AN. 'Test-and-treat': the end of the HIV epidemic? Curr Opin Infect Dis. 2011 Feb;24(1):19-26.
[2] Granich RM, Gilks CF, Dye C, De Cock KM, Williams BG. Universal voluntary HIV testing with immediate antiretroviral therapy as a strategy for elimination of HIV transmission: a mathematical model.Lancet. 2009 Jan 3;373(9657):48-57.
[3] Lissouba P, Taljaard D, Rech D, Dermaux-Msimang V, Legeai C, Lewis D, Singh B, Puren A, Auvert B. Adult male circumcision as an intervention against HIV: an operational study of uptake in a South African community (ANRS 12126). BMC Infect Dis. 2011 Sep 26;11:253

Part 1

Diagnosis and New Technologies

1

Nucleic Acid Testing for HIV-1 Diagnosis and Monitoring

Ricardo Sobhie Diaz
Retrovirology Laboratory Infectious Diseases Division, Paulista School of Medicine, Federal University of Sao Paulo, Medical Director, Laboratório Cento de Genomas, Sao Paulo
Brazil

1. Introduction

In the test and treat era of HIV-1 epidemics, it is becoming extremely urgent to detected HIV-1 infected individuals. It is well known that HIV-1 testing enables health care professions to strategize interventions towards interruption of HIV-1 transmission chains, and to implement antiretroviral therapy. Expanding the number of persons treated with antiretroviral potentially decrease the number of new infections.[1] It is very well determined that the available antibodies based assays are very effective in the majority of cases to detect and confirm HIV-1 infection. However, some exceptions do apply. Diagnosis of HIV-1 infection during the so-called immunologic window period, which is the time between the acquisition of HIV infection and the HIV antibody detection, may be of fundamental importance in some specific cases. It has been debated that effective antiretroviral treatment instituted during acute infection period, which occurs during the immunologic window period, may contribute to a better restructuration of the host immune system, thus allowing to a better long term virologic control or to slower pace of disease progression.[2] Detection of infections during the immunologic window period is also a necessity in order to increase the safety of the blood supply. Furthermore, detection of HIV-1 infection is not specific enough in the cases where the passive transfer of antibodies occurs, such as among infants born from HIV infected mothers. For all these above applications, the direct identification of the pathogen can be an extremely helpful tool, which can be performed using molecular biology based techniques. It is important to bear in mind that passive transfer of antibodies do not occur exclusively among infant born from HIV positive mothers. In one case, a blood recipient from a seropositive unit did not get infected by HIV, but received antibodies that made anti HIV-EIA and Western-blot positive for a period up to six month, being the western blot profile identical to the one found in the infected blood donor.[3] Other case also showed the immediate detection of donors anti-HIV antibodies following a health care work accident, where a broken blood collection tube injured a nurse.[4]

Molecular based techniques area also present in the HIV monitoring tools in tests known as viral load assays. Viral load monitoring can classically predict the pace of HIV-1 disease progression[5] and the effectiveness of antiretroviral treatment. Those tests are still evolving and becoming more sensitive, since detection of low level residual replication is becoming increasingly important in the management of HIV-1 infected individuals. Furthermore, molecular biology has been applied as a valuable tool in detection of HIV strains resistant to antiretrovirals. It is no longer acceptable empirical change in antiretroviral treatment since resistance testing can increase the odds of a successful salvage therapy.[6, 7] As treatment evolves, laboratory tests emerge to make any kind of treatment more effective, safe and predictable. It is the pharmacogenomics playing its role, and again, based in molecular biology techniques. This chapter will describe the challenges related to HIV diagnosis and monitoring, and the contribution of molecular tests in this field.

2. Nucleic acid testing and diagnosis of primary HIV infection

a. Early stages of HIV Infection

After an exposure to HIV-1, and in spite of the exposition route, a dendritic cell will capture the virus and conduct it to the regional lymphonode with the intention of constructing the adaptative immune response.[8] Odds of becoming HIV infected relates to the viral load of the donor of the infection in spite of the rout of HIV transmission. Studies show that there is a threshold level of viral load bellow which heteroseuxual transmission is unlikely to occur.[9, 10] The level of viremia in a blood donor at the time of the donation is the primary factor influencing the probability of the infection.[11] A similar relationship between viral load and HIV transmission has been proposed for perinatal and[12] needlestick exposures.[13, 14] Interestingly however, HIV-1 transmission is considered to be clonal in the large majority of the cases, since 76% start from a single transmitted HIV strains and in 24% of the cases, transmission is seeded by two to five HIV strains.[15] The burst of viremia will start after the dendritic cells reach the regional lymphonode, which takes from 5 to 14 days.[16] Dendridic cells do not get infected by HIV, and after attachment to the DC-SIGN, these cells captures the virus and bring it trapped in its surface or even protected by endocitosis in its way to the regional lymphonode (the dendritic cell present in the genital mucosa is the Langherhan cell). The time elapsed between HIV exposure and the burst of viremia is denominated eclipse period.[17]

When viral replication starts, HIV-1 viral load tends to be exceedingly high, usually with the detection of more than 1 million of HIV RNA copies/mL.[17] Once host immune specific humoral and cellular immunity starts to emerge, viral load tends to decrease to basal values which tend to be constant for the rest for life, and usually affected only by antiretroviral treatment.

Third generation HIV EIA tests can detected HIV as early as 1 month after exposure, and time elapsed between the exposure to HIV and detection of specific antibodies are described as the immunologic window period (Figure 1). The first HIV marker that can be detected is the RNA of virions, which occurs after 17 days (13 to 28), followed by the proviral DNA at the 20th day (18 to 34), followed by the detection of the p24 antigen, which occurs at day 22 (18 to 34).[17] All those markers can be readily used to shorten up the period to detect HIV-1 infection after the exposure event.

b. Nucleic acid testing during the immunologic window period.

The diagnosis of HIV infection is challenging in individuals with recent exposure or symptomatic primary infection, and or the detection of HIV infection from mother to child

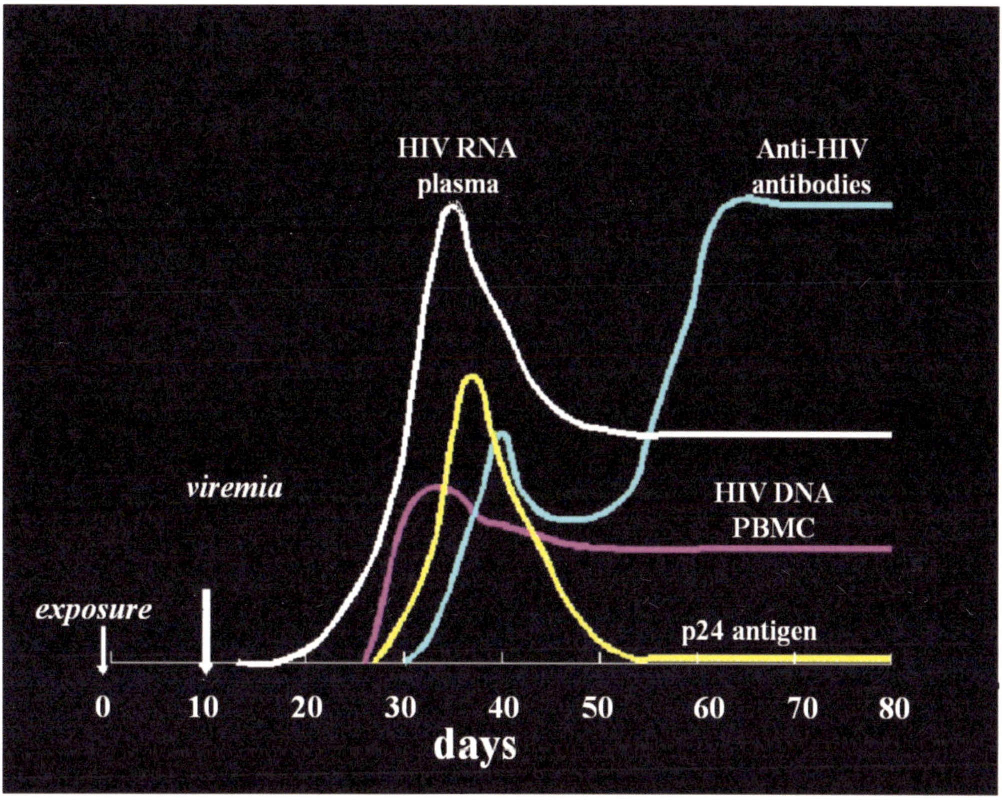

Fig. 1. Approximately sequence and time course of virological and serological events during primary HIV-1 infection. Plasma HIV-1 RNA is detected by commercial viral load assays, whereas HIV DNA in PBMCs is detected by home brew PCE assays.[17]

after vertical exposure. Either of the above mentioned tests, the virion RNA, proviral DNA and p24 antigen can be of utility in the detection of HIV infection after the eclipse period and before fully HIV-1 seroconversion. Especially challenging is the diagnosis among children born from infected mothers. All those children will receive a passive transfer of maternal antibodies which can make anti HIV results positive for up t 18 month after delivery.[18] It is known that the great majority of exposed children will not become HIV infected. Without any sort of antiretroviral prophylaxis, which include the treatment of the mother and use of anitretrovirals by the exposed children for a limited time period, only 20 to 30% of exposed children will become infected.[19] Incident infections will follow to 7% with the use of zidovudine monotherapy by the mothers,[18] being even 50% more efficacious with the use of single doses nevirapine by the time of delivery[20] and to virtually zero if highly active antiretroviral therapy is successfully used, and maintaining maternal viral loads bellow detection limits. Therefore, efforts to overcome the problem of low specificity in diagnosing HIV infection in newborns have been made targeting the direct identification of the virus. The first attempts to overcome this diagnostic problem have been made with the use of co-culture to detected HIV among newborns,[21] which is cumbersome, expensive, takes longer time, and requires well equipped laboratories that cannot be used in large scale in the clinical setting. Therefore, detection of HIV DNA and RNA seems to be more appropriate to detect the vertical transmission of HIV-1.

Timing of vertical HIV transmission is also important in the strategy to test children born from infected mothers. A smaller and variable zproportion of HIV transmission will occur intra-uterus (around 30%), and in these cases, newborns will likely be viremic by the time of birth.[22] In the peripartum transmission, however, the presence of viruses will occur in general around two weeks after birth.[23] Other feature that needs to be taken into account relates to the viral dynamics of HIV- replication among children infected by the vertical route. Whereas among adults, viral load in general reaches the set point by 6 month after HIV infection,[24] and mean basal viral load is inferior to 100,000 RNA copies/mL, children will take much longer to show a week control of viremia after primary infection.[25] In the case of infants, viral loads will be in general above 100,000 RNA copies/mL for a period that is superior to 24 month.[25]

The use of RNA rather than proviral DNA for detection of primary infection has the advantage of providing a shorter window period between HIV acquisition and the first detectable virologic marker, as seen in Figure 1. False positive results with qualitative DNA PCR or quantitative RNA methodologies have been reported in the literature.[26-28] Usually the false positive result can be attributed to the Polymerase Chain reaction (PCR) carry over, decreasing specificity to as low as 96%.[26] As an interesting example, transient HIV-1 infection has been proposed based on the detection of a positive PCR among children who seroreverted (HIV uninfected children born from HIV positive mothers who loose antibodies after 18 month of life).[29] In these cases, detection of human HIV-1 on only one or a few occasions in these infants has been interpreted to indicate that infection may be transient rather than persistent. However, genetic analysis of viruses revealed that either specimens were mistakenly attributed to an infant, or phylogenetic analysis failed to demonstrate the expected linkage between the infant's and the mother's virus,[30] being PCR carry-over the likely explanation for these mistakes.

PCR-carry over, which is a feature of molecular based tests that amplify nucleic acid targets, can be more difficult to be detected in qualitative rather than quantitative assays. In this sense, viral load assays for detecting primary infection has the advantage of potentially discriminating false positive results due to PCR carry over from true positive results since it is expected a high viral load in these situations, being this particularly true for children born from infected mother. In other words, a qualitative assay gives a "yes" or "no" result, whereas the viral load assays can potentially discriminate false positive results since it is expected a very high viral load during primary HIV infection or in infection among children with less than two years old. It has to be taken into account that PCR carry over will always provide a considerable low viral load, which usually is low than 1,000 RNA copies/mL. Therefore, as discussed above, better tests to detect HIV infection in these target populations are assays that targets RNA rather than DNA, and have the quantitative nature rather than qualitative, those tests being the RNA viral load assays. When those tests are performed in children using samples collected after 3 weeks of deliver, the sensitivity, specificity, positive and negative predictive value can be all 100%.[23]

c. HIV-1 RNA quantitation for HIV-1 infection monitoring (ultra-sensitive)

It has been defined since the beginning of the HIV epidemics that HIV-1 viral replication relates well with disease progression and response to treatment.[5] The guidelines for HIV treatment recommend that viral load should be kept as low as possible, preferable bellow detection levels. However, questions have been always related to how sensitive should be a viral load assays. It has been demonstrated that viral replication will occur in spite of the apparently complete HIV suppression using antiretrovirals. One cohort of 130 treated patients kept of HIV-1 RNA viral load bellow 75 copies/mL revealed that 80% of individuals will still present detectable viremia when more sensitive viral load strategies were used (1 RNA copies/mL of plasma) being the median viral load equal 3.1 copies/mL.[31, 32] Other study showed that this low level viremia is likely to be shed by the gastrointestinal tract sanctuary.[33] It has been described that this low level (and sometimes unrecognized) viral replication may lead to a CD4 and CD8+ T cell activation which relates to relates to apoptosis and disease progression.[34, 35] This cell activation can be also detected among elite suppressors, which are individuals that naturally control viremia thus preventing the CD4+ T cell decline, and this cell activation may relate to deleterious aspects among those individuals.[36, 37]

The risk of selecting HIV-1 antiretroviral resistant strains also relates to the level of viral replication, and the pace of emergence of resistant related mutations may be somewhat predictable. Indeed, the number of new mutations relates to the residual viral replication, being directly proportional to the viral load of individuals in virologic failure.[38]

d. HIV-1 antiretrovirals resistance testing

It has been recognized that HIV resistance testing is of benefit in the performance of salvage therapy[7, 31, 39-41] and survival rates.[42] Furthermore, resistant testing exerts great influence in medical decision regarding choice of antiretrovirals in salvage therapy.[43] The current available resistance testing are the so called genotypic resistance tests. Those are indirect measures of resistance, where HIV RNA is obtained, reverse transcribed and cDNA is sequenced to detect the antiretroviral related mutations. Interpretation algorithms are applied to infer the activity of diverse antiretroviral agents. The direct measure of resistance is provided by the phenotypic assays. In these assays, RNA form HIV is also purified and recombinant viruses that have the *pol* gene of patient´s HIV and the backbone of a laboratory virus are produced in vitro. These pseudoviruses are cultured with different concentrations of different antiretrovirals and the resistant related fold change is determined. Fold changes always refer to the amount of drug used to inhibit the patient´s HIV compared to the wild type laboratory strain. Biological and clinical cut-offs are used to infer the probability of response to specific antiretrovirals. Genotypic tests are easier to perform, more available and less expensive than phenotypic based assays. They also are more sensitive in detecting resistance when mixtures of mutant and wild type viruses are present, since it is likely that resistant strains will be overwhelmed by the more fit wild type strains in the initial culture producing the pseudoviruses.[44] The quantitative nature of phenotypic based assays may be of utility in analyzing the highly resistance strains. Phenotypic tests are also advantageous for new antiretrovirals with poorly defined resistance profile and perhaps for non-B strains, where resistance pathways and mutations may not be yet available. Furthermore, the presence of fold change and clinical cut-off increase the confidence of physicians in the choice of salvage therapy.[43] There is also the virtual phenotype test, which is in fact a genotypic based assays. In these tests, HIV-1 *pol* sequences are submitted to a specific database, which will infer the phenotypic profile of viruses providing fold changes and clinical cut-offs. In fact, performance of virtual phenotype has been comparable or better than the performance found using phenotype for salvage therapy.[41, 45] The likely explanation for the alleged better performance of virtual phenotype as compared to the "real" phenotype relies in the fact that virtual phenotype will be less likely to underestimate resistance since mixtures of wild type and resistant strains found in the sequencing process will be considered as resistant. Conversely, as explained above, mixtures of wild type/resistant will facilitate overgrow of wild type strains in cell culture.

e. HIV-1 Tropism

The practical issue of HIV-1 tropism emerged with the development of CCR5 antagonists as antiretrovirals. Nonetheless, HIV tropism has been studied for a long time in the attempt to correlate the HIV-1 correceptor use with cytopathycity. In summary, HIV may use CCR5 and CXCR4 chemokine receptors for entry, and viruses that exclusively use the CCR5 are denominated R5, viruses that use CXCR4 are X4, whereas viruses able to use both coreceptors are dual tropic (reviewed by Moore et al).[16] Infection usually starts with R5 viruses and as HIV-1 quasispecies evolves, CXCR4 using strains may emerge. There is also the association between the emergence of CXCR4 using strains and rapid HIV-1 disease progression.[46] Therefore, it is conceivable that the determination and monitoring HIV-1 tropism over time may be of use in the decision of introduction of antiretroviral treatment or more frequent evaluation of CD4+ T cell levels in the infected patient.

The main utility of tropism determination relates to the decision of use of CCR5 antagonists such as maraviroc, since this specific class of antiretrovirals will lose activity in the presence of detectable X4 or dual tropic viruses.[47] Therefore, a tropism test before treatment with these drugs is required; gold standard tropism tests being the phenotypic based tests. One phenotypic tropism test constructs pseudoviruses containing the gp160 of patient's viruses and a backbone of HIV-1 laboratory virus plus the luciferase gene.[48] Two lineages of cells containing either the CCR5 or the CXCR4 coreceptors are used in two distinct lab reactions. Once infected, light will be generated from cells due the presence of the luciferase gene, and HIV can be detected in the culture either inside cells harboring CCR5 and/or CXCR4 coreceptors. If HIV is detected only in the culture of cells harboring CCR5 coreceptor, viruses will be classified as R5, whereas X4 viruses will appear only in the culture of cells harboring CXCR4 coreceptors. In the case viruses are detected in both cultures, it is reported that dual mixed and/or mixtures of R5 and X4 are present. Alternatively, genotropism tests can be used. These tests detect substitutions at the V3 region of gp120 HIV-1 gene in order to predict the CXCR4 use by viruses present in the patient's quaispecie. Although phenotypic and genotypic tests do not fully agree with each other, genotypic tests are probably equally able to predict virologic treatment failure in maraviroc containing antiretroviral schemes[47] and have been advocate as preferential in some guidelines.[49]

3. References

[1] Montaner, J.S., *Treatment as prevention--a double hat-trick.* Lancet, 2011. 378(9787): p. 208-9.

[2] Cellerai, C., et al., *Proliferation capacity and cytotoxic activity are mediated by functionally and phenotypically distinct virus-specific CD8 T cells defined by interleukin-7R{alpha} (CD127) and perforin expression.* J Virol, 2010. 84(8): p. 3868-78.

[3] Salomao, R., et al., *Passive transfer of HIV-1 antibodies and absence of HIV infection after the transfusion of HIV-1-seropositive red cells.* Transfusion, 2000. 40(2): p. 252-3.

[4] deOliveira CF, D.R., Harmache A, Frenkel LM, Gupta P, Learn GH, Mullins JI, Busch MP., *Passive transfer of HIV Antibodies Following a Health Care Worker (HCW) Accident, and Transmission of HIV-1 Antiretroviral Resistant Strain: Implications for HCW Post-Exposure Management.* American Journal of Infectious Diseases, 2008. 4 ((4)): p. 244-256.

[5] Mellors, J.W., et al., *Plasma viral load and CD4+ lymphocytes as prognostic markers of HIV-1 infection.* Ann Intern Med, 1997. 126(12): p. 946-54.

[6] Palella, F.J., Jr., et al., *Declining morbidity and mortality among patients with advanced human immunodeficiency virus infection. HIV Outpatient Study Investigators.* N Engl J Med, 1998. 338(13): p. 853-60.

[7] Tural, C., et al., *Clinical utility of HIV-1 genotyping and expert advice: the Havana trial.* AIDS, 2002. 16(2): p. 209-18.

[8] Kawamura, T., et al., *R5 HIV productively infects Langerhans cells, and infection levels are regulated by compound CCR5 polymorphisms.* Proc Natl Acad Sci U S A, 2003. 100(14): p. 8401-6.

[9] Operskalski, E.A., et al., *Role of viral load in heterosexual transmission of human immunodeficiency virus type 1 by blood transfusion recipients. Transfusion Safety Study Group.* Am J Epidemiol, 1997. 146(8): p. 655-61.

[10] Lee, T.H., et al., *Absence of HIV-1 DNA in high-risk seronegative individuals using high-input polymerase chain reaction.* AIDS, 1991. 5(10): p. 1201-7.

[11] Busch, M.P., et al., *Factors influencing human immunodeficiency virus type 1 transmission by blood transfusion. Transfusion Safety Study Group.* J Infect Dis, 1996. 174(1): p. 26-33.

[12] Wilfert, C.M., et al., *Pathogenesis of pediatric human immunodeficiency virus type 1 infection.* J Infect Dis, 1994. 170(2): p. 286-92.

[13] Gerberding, J.L., *Incidence and prevalence of human immunodeficiency virus, hepatitis B virus, hepatitis C virus, and cytomegalovirus among health care personnel at risk for blood exposure: final report from a longitudinal study.* J Infect Dis, 1994. 170(6): p. 1410-7.

[14] Cardo, D.M., et al., *A case-control study of HIV seroconversion in health care workers after percutaneous exposure. Centers for Disease Control and Prevention Needlestick Surveillance Group.* N Engl J Med, 1997. 337(21): p. 1485-90.

[15] Keele, B.F., et al., *Identification and characterization of transmitted and early founder virus envelopes in primary HIV-1 infection.* Proc Natl Acad Sci U S A, 2008. 105(21): p. 7552-7.

[16] Moore, J.P., et al., *The CCR5 and CXCR4 coreceptors--central to understanding the transmission and pathogenesis of human immunodeficiency virus type 1 infection.* AIDS Res Hum Retroviruses, 2004. 20(1): p. 111-26.

[17] Lee, H.Y., et al., *Modeling sequence evolution in acute HIV-1 infection.* J Theor Biol, 2009. 261(2): p. 341-60.

[18] Connor, E.M., et al., *Reduction of maternal-infant transmission of human immunodeficiency virus type 1 with zidovudine treatment. Pediatric AIDS Clinical Trials Group Protocol 076 Study Group.* N Engl J Med, 1994. 331(18): p. 1173-80.

[19] *Rates of mother-to-child transmission of HIV-1 in Africa, America, and Europe: results from 13 perinatal studies. The Working Group on Mother-To-Child Transmission of HIV.* J Acquir Immune Defic Syndr Hum Retrovirol, 1995. 8(5): p. 506-10.

[20] Guay, L.A., et al., *Intrapartum and neonatal single-dose nevirapine compared with zidovudine for prevention of mother-to-child transmission of HIV-1 in Kampala, Uganda: HIVNET 012 randomised trial.* Lancet, 1999. 354(9181): p. 795-802.

[21] Paul, M.O., et al., *Laboratory diagnosis of infection status in infants perinatally exposed to human immunodeficiency virus type 1.* J Infect Dis, 1996. 173(1): p. 68-76.

[22] Nourse, C.B. and K.M. Butler, *Perinatal transmission of HIV and diagnosis of HIV infection in infants: a review.* Ir J Med Sci, 1998. 167(1): p. 28-32.

[23] Souza, I.E., et al., *RNA viral load test for early diagnosis of vertical transmission of HIV-1 infection.* J Acquir Immune Defic Syndr, 2000. 23(4): p. 358-60.

[24] Vidal, C., et al., *Lack of evidence of a stable viral load set-point in early stage asymptomatic patients with chronic HIV-1 infection.* AIDS, 1998. 12(11): p. 1285-9.

[25] Shearer, W.T., et al., *Viral load and disease progression in infants infected with human immunodeficiency virus type 1. Women and Infants Transmission Study Group.* N Engl J Med, 1997. 336(19): p. 1337-42.

[26] Cunningham, C.K., et al., *Comparison of human immunodeficiency virus 1 DNA polymerase chain reaction and qualitative and quantitative RNA polymerase chain reaction in human immunodeficiency virus 1-exposed infants.* Pediatr Infect Dis J, 1999. 18(1): p. 30-5.

[27] de Mendoza, C., A. Holguin, and V. Soriano, *False positives for HIV using commercial viral load quantification assays.* AIDS, 1998. 12(15): p. 2076-7.

[28] Long, S.S. and H.W. Lischner, *Early and accurate detection of infection with human immunodeficiency virus type 1 in vertically exposed infants.* J Pediatr, 1996. 129(2): p. 189-90.

[29] Bryson, Y.J., et al., *Clearance of HIV infection in a perinatally infected infant.* N Engl J Med, 1995. 332(13): p. 833-8.

[30] Frenkel, L.M., et al., *Genetic evaluation of suspected cases of transient HIV-1 infection of infants.* Science, 1998. 280(5366): p. 1073-7.
[31] Maldarelli, F., et al., *ART suppresses plasma HIV-1 RNA to a stable set point predicted by pretherapy viremia.* PLoS Pathog, 2007. 3(4): p. e46.
[32] Palmer, S., et al., *Low-level viremia persists for at least 7 years in patients on suppressive antiretroviral therapy.* Proc Natl Acad Sci U S A, 2008. 105(10): p. 3879-84.
[33] Anton, P.A., et al., *Multiple measures of HIV burden in blood and tissue are correlated with each other but not with clinical parameters in aviremic subjects.* AIDS, 2003. 17(1): p. 53-63.
[34] Hunt, P.W., et al., *The independent effect of drug resistance on T cell activation in HIV infection.* AIDS, 2006. 20(5): p. 691-9.
[35] Holm, G.H. and D. Gabuzda, *Distinct mechanisms of CD4+ and CD8+ T-cell activation and bystander apoptosis induced by human immunodeficiency virus type 1 virions.* J Virol, 2005. 79(10): p. 6299-311.
[36] Owen, R.E., et al., *HIV+ elite controllers have low HIV-specific T-cell activation yet maintain strong, polyfunctional T-cell responses.* AIDS. 24(8): p. 1095-105.
[37] Sodora, D.L. and G. Silvestri, *Immune activation and AIDS pathogenesis.* AIDS, 2008. 22(4): p. 439-46.
[38] Napravnik, S., et al., *HIV-1 drug resistance evolution among patients on potent combination antiretroviral therapy with detectable viremia.* J Acquir Immune Defic Syndr, 2005. 40(1): p. 34-40.
[39] Durant, J., et al., *Drug-resistance genotyping in HIV-1 therapy: the VIRADAPT randomised controlled trial.* Lancet, 1999. 353(9171): p. 2195-9.
[40] Cohen, C.J., et al., *A randomized trial assessing the impact of phenotypic resistance testing on antiretroviral therapy.* AIDS, 2002. 16(4): p. 579-88.
[41] Perez-Elias, M.J., et al., *Phenotype or virtual phenotype for choosing antiretroviral therapy after failure: a prospective, randomized study.* Antivir Ther, 2003. 8(6): p. 577-84.
[42] Palella, F.J., Jr., et al., *The association of HIV susceptibility testing with survival among HIV-infected patients receiving antiretroviral therapy: a cohort study.* Ann Intern Med, 2009. 151(2): p. 73-84.
[43] Diaz, R.S., et al., *HIV-1 resistance testing influences treatment decision-making.* Braz J Infect Dis. 14(5): p. 489-94.
[44] Andreoni, M., *Viral phenotype and fitness.* New Microbiol, 2004. 27(2 Suppl 1): p. 71-6.
[45] Mazzotta, F., et al., *Real versus virtual phenotype to guide treatment in heavily pretreated patients: 48-week follow-up of the Genotipo-Fenotipo di Resistenza (GenPheRex) trial.* J Acquir Immune Defic Syndr, 2003. 32(3): p. 268-80.
[46] Koot, M., et al., *Prognostic value of HIV-1 syncytium-inducing phenotype for rate of CD4+ cell depletion and progression to AIDS.* Ann Intern Med, 1993. 118(9): p. 681-8.
[47] McGovern, R.A., et al., *Population-based V3 genotypic tropism assay: a retrospective analysis using screening samples from the A4001029 and MOTIVATE studies.* AIDS. 24(16): p. 2517-25.
[48] Whitcomb, J.M., et al., *Development and characterization of a novel single-cycle recombinant-virus assay to determine human immunodeficiency virus type 1 coreceptor tropism.* Antimicrob Agents Chemother, 2007. 51(2): p. 566-75.

[49] Vandekerckhove, L.P., et al., *European guidelines on the clinical management of HIV-1 tropism testing*. Lancet Infect Dis. 11(5): p. 394-407.

2

HIV-2: Testing Specificities

Jean P. Ruelle
UCLouvain, AIDS Reference Laboratory
Belgium

1. Introduction

1.1 Discovery of HIV-2: A story of antibody reactivity

Two years after the isolation of the first AIDS virus in 1983 (Barre-Sinoussi et al. 1983), a simian virus inducing a similar pathology was described in rhesus monkeys in captivity (Letvin et al. 1985). Apparently healthy individuals living in Senegal had antibodies that reacted better with the antigens of the simian virus than with those from the human virus (Barin et al. 1985). At the same period, two patients originating from West Africa were hospitalized in France and in Portugal with typical symptoms of AIDS, whereas their serology was negative for the human virus now called HIV-1. The second virus causing AIDS was isolated in 1986 (Clavel et al. 1986). It was then described in various countries of West Africa, and was later called Human immunodeficiency virus type 2 (HIV-2) (Brun-Vezinet et al. 1987; Clavel et al. 1987). It is classified in the *Retroviridae* family within the *lentivirus* genus. Among the lentiviruses, the two HIV are phylogenetically closer to simian lentiviruses than those infecting other animal species, explaining the antibody cross-reactivity observed at first (Chakrabarti et al. 1987). The HIV-2 genome is closest to SIVsm infecting sooty mangabeys (Hirsch et al. 1989), whereas HIV-1 is closest to SIVcpz infecting chimpanzees (Huet et al. 1990).

1.2 Clinical outcome

HIV-2 differs from HIV-1 in its lower rate of disease progression and infectivity (Jaffar et al. 2004). The routes of transmission are identical to those described for HIV-1, but with lower rates for both horizontal and vertical transmissions, and correlate with the mean lower viral load in HIV-2 infected patients (O'Donovan et al. 2000). The majority of them are long-term non-progressors (LTNP), meaning that they don't develop symptoms and that the infection does not significantly affect their survival (Rowland-Jones & Whittle 2007). Nevertheless, patients experiencing disease progression and AIDS share the same likelihood of morbidity and mortality as seen in HIV-1 infection (Schim van der Loeff et al. 2002), and will be eligible for antiretroviral therapy. AIDS-defining events are comparable in both types of infections (Martinez-Steele et al. 2007). The distinction between LTNP, patients who remain asymptomatic for at least 8 years while CD4 counts are above 500 cells/ul, and controllers, who control HIV replication without therapy, was recently analysed in the French ANRS cohort; they represented respectively 6.1% and 9.1% (Thiébaut et al. 2011). Although those low percentages contrast with previous publications, it remains clear that LTNP in HIV-2 are far most frequent compared to HIV-1 cohorts, and that low viral load is the main feature of non-progression. Cellular immunity and the maintenance of early-differentiated $CD8^+$ T-cells contribute to low immune activation and low viral replication (Leligdowicz et al. 2010). Understanding the mechanisms underlying HIV-2 biology and the immune response, as a model for attenuated-HIV disease, are important in the concept of HIV vaccines (Leligdowicz & Rowland-Jones 2008).

1.3 Sensitivity to ARV drugs

HIV-2 is naturally resistant to non-nucleosidic reverse transcriptase inhibitors, including those of second generation, and to the fusion inhibitor enfuvirtide (Witvrouw et al. 2004; Andries et al. 2004; Poveda et al. 2004). The sensitivity to some protease inhibitors is reduced: amprenavir and its prodrug are not active, and contradictory results were published for atazanavir and tipranavir (Desbois et al. 2008; Brower et al. 2008). Moreover, the genetic barrier to resistance is reduced for several NRTIs and PIs (Smith et al. 2009). In the context of that reduced therapeutic arsenal, recent drug classes represent welcome options.

Theoretically, CCR-5 antagonists can be used to treat HIV-2 infection, but two main issues need to be solved: no tropism assay is currently available for clinical routine, and the possible impact of the broader co-receptor usage compared to HIV-1 is not known (Calado et al. 2010). Nevertheless some experimental case studies showed treatment success (Armstrong-James et al. 2010).

Integrase inhibitors are active on HIV-2; several *in vitro* studies on patient isolates and case series showed good activity (Roquebert et al. 2008; Damond et al. 2008a): raltegravir is therefore an option in case of failure or intolerability to other drugs (Francisci et al. 2011), but long-term data are lacking at this point (Gottlieb et al. 2011). No randomized clinical trials were performed to investigate response to treatment in HIV-2 patients (Gottlieb et al. 2008a). Data on treatment efficacy are obtained through cohort analysis, case series or collaborative networking between cohorts: a double-NRTI backbone combined to a boosted-PI is the preferred first-line regimen (Benard et al. 2011). Therapy limitations underline the importance of an accurate diagnosis of HIV-2 infection, particularly in countries where drug classes availability is limited (Peterson et al. 2011).

1.4 Epidemiology

The evaluation of the total number of case varies between 1 and 2 million infected people worldwide, the majority living in West African countries (Gottlieb et al. 2008a). The highest prevalence was noticed in Guinea-Bissau around 1990, where 17% of blood donors were positive (Poulsen et al. 1993; Naucler et al. 1989). Since then, the HIV-2 prevalence has declined, and is nowadays lower than 1% in the global population in most countries, with the exceptions of the Gambia, Guinea-Bissau and Côte d'Ivoire (da Silva et al. 2008; Sangare et al. 1998). The prevalence of HIV-1 infection has increased during the last two decades in West Africa, and has now exceeds that of type 2 (van Tienen et al. 2010). Although declining, HIV-2 remains of concern particularly in urban areas. The prevalence is more important in older groups, above 45 years of age (van Tienen et al. 2010). Outside West Africa, the virus is present in European countries, essentially in Portugal and France who share colonial histories with endemic regions (Valadas et al. 2009; Barin et al. 2007). Sporadic cases are found in other African and European countries, in Brazil, in the Middle East, in Japan, Korea and in India. The majority of patients in these countries were born in or had a possible transmission link with West Africa (Campbell-Yesufu & Gandhi 2011). The virus is very rare in North America (Torian et al. 2010; Centers for Disease Control 2011).

1.5 Diversity of HIV-2: Origins and impact on laboratory assays

Eight groups of HIV-2 have been described, named A to H (Damond et al. 2004). Each of those phylogenetically distinct groups corresponds to a cross-species transmission from monkey to man (Sharp et al. 2001). Only groups A and B spread in the human population while other groups seem epidemic dead-ends possibly because of weak adaptation to the human organism (Gao et al. 1994). A/B recombinant forms appeared (Yamaguchi et al. 2008) and disseminated outside West Africa (Ibe et al. 2010). Based on HIV-2 sequences with available sampling dates, the date of the most recent common ancestor was inferred by phylogeny: group A and B strains appeared respectively around 1940 and 1945 (Lemey et al. 2003). Molecular clock analysis favours the hypothesis of a zoonotic transmission during the first half of the 20th century, followed by an epidemic dissemination during the 1960s. The independence war of Guinea-Bissau between 1963 and 1974 offered the circumstances favouring human transmissions (Poulsen et al. 2000; Gomes et al. 2003). Genetic variability between HIV-2 groups, and between strains of the same group is important. The most conserved genomic regions are the LTRs, followed by the *gag* and *pol* genes (Kanki 1991). Several examples in the next paragraphs will illustrate the impact of viral diversity on laboratory assays: the use of conserved epitopes can lead to cross-reactivity between HIV types in serology. On the opposite, if an assay targets particularly variable regions, the probability of a false negative result or an underestimated quantification will rise. Serological screening and confirmatory assays, as well as nucleic acid tests (NAT) used for diagnosis or clinical follow-up, must thus take into account HIV-2 diversity from design through field validation.

2. Diagnosis of HIV-2 infection

2.1 Screening assays

The diagnosis of HIV-1 or -2 infection is based on serology, mostly using enzyme immunoassays (EIA). As antibodies appear in the serum several weeks post-infection, antibody detection was progressively improved in order to reduce the window period between infection and test positivity. Sensitive assays detecting IgM and IgG are positive a mean of 3 weeks after transmission. Fourth generation assays sensitive to both HIV-antigen and anti-HIV antibodies, also called "combo-tests", are able to detect an acute infection as early as 2 weeks after the transmission event, when the viral replication level is extremely high (review in Branson 2010). The duration of the window period was established for HIV-1 infections and is largely unknown for HIV-2. A study on recent seroconverters showed that viral loads are on average 28-fold times lower compared to HIV-1 (Andersson et al. 2000). As replication capacity is lower and viral turnover slower, there exists the possibility that the time between HIV-2 infection and seropositivity is longer.

Initially designed for the detection of HIV-1 group M, most commercial tests are nowadays reactive to anti-HIV-2 and anti-HIV-1 group O antibodies, but not all of them. As disease progression is on the mean slower in HIV-2 and that the majority of patients are asymptomatic, we can expect to underdiagnose HIV-2 infection in countries or regions where HIV screening assays do not recognize anti-HIV-2 antibodies. It is therefore recommended to opt for tests sensitive to anti-HIV-1 and -2. For antigen detection, fourth generation assays reacting with HIV-1 p24 Ag have no specific component to detect HIV-2 antigens. However, because of conserved regions in the Gag capsid protein and its epitopes, p24-sensitive antigen assays can detect the HIV-2 related antigen, the p26. We cannot exclude a difference of sensitivity for HIV-2 antigen detection in HIV combo assays. That difference has probably a negligible impact in clinical practice, because the probability to test a patient in early acute HIV-2 infection is very low. Nevertheless, as for HIV-1 infection, in the presence of an HIV negative test and clinical signs or seroconversion illness, the patient should be retested 2 to 4 weeks later (Poljak et al. 2009). If a risky behaviour is suspected in an HIV-2 prevalent area, a period of 3 months is recommended to ascertain the negativity.

Several rapid tests using immunoprecipitation techniques for antibody detection are approved for clinical use, using serum, whole blood or saliva. As the result can be obtained in 20 minutes, it may be appropriate for the screening of individuals who may not return for the results in conventional settings. They require a minimum of reagents and infrastructure: their use is widespread in resource-constrained countries, in point-of-care facilities, or in centres for voluntary testing. Rapid assays of four generation are currently developed, such as Alere Determine HIV1/2 combo assay (Inverness Medical, UK). Although its performance for antibody detection is comparable to reference EIA, the assay's antigen sensitivity is weaker than references and is unable to detect HIV-2 antigens (Beelaert & Fransen 2010).

Antibody screening assays relying on other methods than EIA or immunoprecipitation are currently in development, with the goal to enhance specificity and to have a higher throughput (Talha et al. 2011).

Present day screening assays have an excellent sensitivity close to 100%, and a specificity higher than 99%. Their negative predictive value is very high, but the positive predictive value is low, depending on the local prevalence. False positive results are thus common in practice, and a second independent test should be used to confirm the initial result. As the first-line assays give a positive signal in screening whether due to anti-HIV-1 or anti-HIV-2 antibodies, confirmatory tests used in clinical settings should be able to discriminate the type of virus and arrive to the final diagnosis of HIV-2 infection.

2.2 Discrimination of anti-HIV-2 antibodies

Three types of assays are widespread in clinical laboratories for the discrimination of HIV type by serology: Western Blots, line immunoassays, and rapid tests. Commercial Western blot registered for diagnostics such as New LAV Blot II (Bio-Rad, CA) or HIV Blot 1.2 WB (Genelabs, CA) use immobilised HIV antigens to detect specific IgG antibodies to different viral proteins. A result is interpreted as positive if bands reveal a reaction with two or more of the following HIV antigens: p24, gp41, or gp120/160. The result is considered as indeterminate if bands are present, but fewer than two reacting with the antigens cited above. Western blot has several pitfalls. It can overestimate HIV-2 infection, particularly in regions with very low prevalence, because of frequent cross-reactions (Qiu et al. 2009; McKellar et al. 2008). Moreover, the turnaround time is higher compared to line immunoassay or rapid tests, it needs more laboratory material, and generates more waste.

The use of a commercial line peptide assay such as Inno-Lia (InnoGenetics, Belgium) engineered with synthetic peptides, allows more standardised results and gives less significant cross reactivity for the discrimination between type 1 and 2 infections (Amor et al. 2009).

The rapid test Genie HIV-1/HIV-2 (Bio-Rad, CA) is a test based on the immunochromatography principle for the specific detection and differentiation of HIV-1 and HIV-2 antibodies. In several West African countries, national algorithms are based on rapid tests including Genie I/II (Kania et al. 2010). Double reactive samples as defined in Burkina Faso were retested with line peptide assay: only 59% of dually reactive serums had concordant results. Among dual positive samples, 15 % had a detectable HIV-2 plasma viral load while 60% of HIV-2 seropositive patients had a detectable viraemia (Ruelle et al. 2007).

Double HIV-1/HIV-2 infections are thus largely overestimated. Double-reactive samples in serology tested with specific qualitative PCRs confirmed only 32% of double infections (Ciccaglione et al. 2010). The group of HIV-2 may also influence serological cross-reactivity: a strong reaction was described between group B and HIV-1 *env* antigen, mostly in the gp transmembrane glycoprotein (Damond et al. 2001a).

2.3 Nucleic acid tests (NAT)

Molecular tests are available for the quantitative detection of HIV-1 plasma RNA, beside commercial plasma viral load assays. No commercial qualitative or quantitative test is available for HIV-2. Several in-house methods have been published and validated (Schutten et al. 2000; Ruelle et al. 2004; Damond et al. 2001b; Ferns & Garson 2006), but are restricted to specialised laboratory. As many HIV-2 patients has very low plasma viral load, without any ARV therapy, RNA counts will often fall under the PCR limit of detection. As a consequence, the viraemia can often not be considered as a diagnostic marker.

However, proviral DNA can be theoretically detected in all HIV-2 seropositive patients, at least if the PCR is sensitive enough, and if the primers target a sufficiently conserved region. The amount of DNA present in PBMC was thought to be similar to that in HIV-1 infection. It seems to be the case in patients experiencing low CD4 counts, but can be lower for controllers (Gueudin et al. 2008; Gottlieb, Hawes et al. 2008). Globally the ratio plasma RNA/proviral DNA is lower in HIV-2 infection, due to putative differences in the replicative cycle. It is estimated that HIV proviral DNA is present in 1 cell out of 10,000 PBMC. Laboratory NAT protocols should therefore use a sufficient number of cells to avoid false negative PCR results: to detect 10 HIV DNA copies, we should introduce in the PCR reaction a DNA volume corresponding to the extraction of a minimum of 100,000 cells.

2.4 Proposed HIV-2 testing algorithm

A decisional algorithm is shown in Figure 1; it avoids the shortcomings of Western Blot detailed above, allows differentiating HIV-2 from HIV-1 upon confirmation, and reduces the window period in case of acute infection. When a confirmatory test gives an HIV untypable

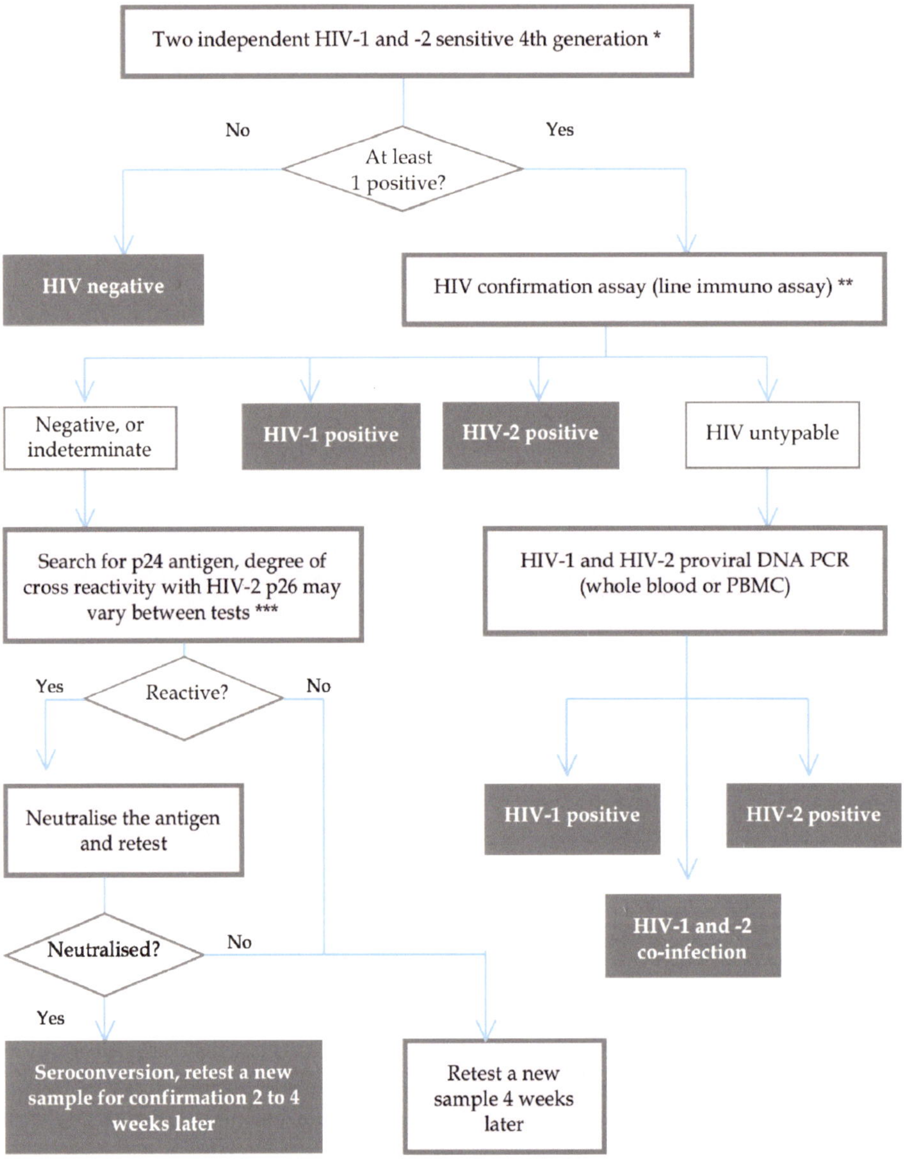

* Alternatively one single test if high HIV prevalence
** Alternatively a rapid test discriminant for HIV type
*** If not available, retest a new sample 2 to 4 weeks later. Not informative about HIV type in case of positivity

Fig. 1. Algorithm for HIV-2 confirmation

result, we should consider a NAT amplifying specifically HIV-2 proviral DNA. A single or dual-infection result will strongly influence the therapeutic management, as recommended first-line therapies are based on NNRTI in most countries. Although no study is available, the proviral DNA approach in case of dual-reactivity should be cost-effective by avoiding therapeutic failures.

2.5 Children born to HIV-2 seropositive mothers

Vertical transmission occurs rarely, reported rates vary between 0.1 and 2% (Burgard et al. 2010; Padua et al. 2009). Undetectable viral load during the third trimester of pregnancy and at delivery is a good predictor of prevention success. Due to passive transfer of maternal antibodies, the diagnosis of a mother-to-child HIV transmission is based on viral genome amplification. In addition to the issues of low DNA amount and primer mismatches discussed above for provirus detection, viral turnover is lower in HIV-2 infection and we have virtually no data on what occurs after the child's infection. Plasma RNA should be amplified in parallel with proviral DNA, or alternatively different sets of primers should be used to amplify the same DNA sample. As viral genetic variability can be responsible of PCR failure (Padua et al. 2009), some authors recommend amplifying one sample from the mother, with the same sets of primers, as a positive control. Ideally, the follow-up of the baby should include the search for proviral DNA: if viral genome is not detected at the age of 3 months, vertical transmission did not occur. In countries where NATs are not available, prevention with antiretroviral therapy including PIs will considerably reduce the chances of transmission.

3. Plasma viral load

3.1 Available assays and standardisation

Plasma viral load correspond to the number of RNA genomes present in the patient's blood, expressed in copies per millilitre (ml) of plasma or in log copies/ml. It is a predictor of disease progression: viral replication will enhance CD4 count drop (Gottlieb et al. 2002). RNA quantification also allows the identification of HIV-2 controllers.

No commercial assay was approved for HIV-2 viral load monitoring in clinical settings. Some companies developed PCR primers sets, other offer a biochemical assay based on reverse transcriptase activity, but no major HIV-1 viral load platform has a version dedicated to HIV-2. Some studies described the use of the Nuclisens HIV-1 assay (Biomérieux, France), an isothermal RNA amplifiction method, applied to HIV-2 group A (Rodes et al. 2007). When compared to in-house RT-PCR assays, sensitivity was not optimal (Damond et al. 2008b).

Plasma viral load assays are mainly restricted to some reference laboratories across Europe, and in some African centres. Real-time PCR is by far the most common technology used by those laboratories. If the coverage is sufficient for the HIV-2 cohorts in Europe, most West African countries lack reliable assays to monitor their patients.

RNA quantification is ensured by an external standard curve in PCR. Several methods were published using an electron microscopy counted reference strain. The main advantages of such standard is that the process of extraction and amplification is exactly the same as a sample, avoiding extraction yield discrepancies, and that one quantified stock conserved in aliquots at -80°C can be used for a long period of time. As a drawback, the viral load is expressed in RNA genomes per ml and not in viral particles: some non-infectious virions present in a viral stock do not contain nucleic acid and can therefore bias the result. As an example, if 1000 viral particles contain less than the 2000 supposed genome copies, the standard will be too high and the samples tested will be under-quantified. Another option is the use of nucleic acids quantified by spectrophotometry as standards. The count of RNA standards is more close to the real number of genome copies than counted particles, but RNAs are less stable and can easily be degraded by environmental RNAse or by too long conservation periods. Moreover, a supplementary control on the extraction step must be added to the assay, and traces of parental DNA serving as template for RNA synthesis can also bias the RNA quantification.

The quality and reproducibility of HIV-2 viral load assays was evaluated across Europe and in the Gambia through the AcHIeV$_2$e collaborative network (Damond et al. 2008b). A first round showed that most of the assays gave reproducible results, but important discrepancies were seen for absolute quantifications. As those were possibly linked to the use of different standards, a second round of controls was sent around together with one aliquot of counted particles. Inter-laboratory homogeneity was then better, and primer mismatches were suspected as the origin of result variability (Damond et al. 2011). A good correlation of results was obtained for HIV-2 group A samples, but quantification of group B strains is extremely variable between laboratories. The latter evaluations underscore the need of a common standard if multi-centric assessments using viral load as a parameter are foreseen, and the need for an enhanced quality for HIV-2 group B quantifications. Two reference standards are now available, made respectively from strains ROD and CAM, belonging to group A. Their titres are expressed in international units (IU), which raises the unsolved issue about the use of IU vs. RNA copies in HIV clinical practice.

3.2 Indications and interpretation

Plasma viral load is indicated to monitor the absence or degree of viral replication during antiretroviral therapy. If we hypothesise that HIV-2 patients in need of therapy have the same likelihood to progress as compared to HIV-1, we can assume that recommendations for the follow-up are the same: viral load measurement at therapy initiation, one month after and then every 3 months, with the goal of achieving durable suppression. In resource-constraint settings, clinical monitoring alone should be used to expand antiretroviral therapy, although it is not the optimal solution (Laurent et al. 2011). Given the mean slower disease progression and the high proportion of non-progressors, the monitoring of HIV-2 viral load could be spaced for untreated patients from 6 months to 1 year, but no study support clearly that recommendation until now. In case CD4 counts drop or if disease progresses despite an undetectable viral load, the plasma should be retested with an alternative assay to avoid a possible problem of genetic variability (Gilleece et al. 2010).

4. Resistance testing

4.1 Genotypic assays

To determine the sensitivity of an HIV-1 isolate to antiretroviral drugs, genotypic assays are the most widespread in clinical laboratories by sequencing the viral gene coding for the drug target (protease, reverse transcriptase, integrase and envelope glycoproteins). The translated amino acid sequence is compared to that of a reference strain to establish a list of mutations. From that list, sensitivity to each drug is inferred by interpretation rules. Although some phenotypic assays can be used in the clinic, their use is restricted by much higher costs, the need for a biosafety level 3 laboratory, and higher turnaround times; they are usually developed for research purposes. Alternatively, virtual HIV-1 phenotypes are available, translating genotypic data into IC_{50} fold changes and activity cut-offs (review in Schutten 2006). Clinically relevant cut-offs were inferred using clinical trials and cohort data (Winters et al. 2008).

None of the commercial assays available for HIV-1 resistance testing can be used for HIV-2: resistance assays are restricted to some reference laboratories, mostly in Europe, and rely on home-brew protocols. Classically Sanger sequencing is performed after RT-PCR amplification from plasma RNA: sensitive PCR protocols are needed, as HIV-2 viral loads are low. Next-generation sequencing allowing detection of more variants in quasi-species would help to understand HIV-2 specific viral dynamics and resistance pathways.

4.2 Interpretation rules

Even if the two types of HIV share some major resistance mutations, the genetic barrier, the pathways leading to resistance and the frequency of mutations differ (Ntemgwa et al. 2009; Smith et al. 2009). Therefore the interpretation rules developed to determine HIV-1 resistance do not apply to HIV-2. Some natural polymorphisms in the HIV-2 *pol* gene correspond to resistance mutations in HIV-1 algorithms (Bercoff et al. 2010; Rodes et al. 2006; Colson et al. 2005). Compared to HIV-1, the RT multi-drug resistance mutation Q151M is far more frequent after therapy failure, as the K65R mutation (Descamps et al. 2004). Two sets of HIV-2 specific interpretation rules have been published so far: the ANRS (Agence Nationale de Recherche sur le SIDA et les Hépatites, Paris, France) and the Rega (Rega Institute, KULeuven, Belgium) rules. The latest versions of those algorithms are available on line (ANRS-AC11 2011; Gomes et al. 2009). The first one is more specific, as the list includes only mutations for which the impact was clearly demonstrated in several publications: K65R, Q151M, M184V and S215 changes in the RT (Damond et al. 2005), as well as mutations at positions 143, 148 and 155 in the integrase (Charpentier et al. 2011). The second algorithm is probably more sensitive as the list includes other minor mutations for which an impact has been described, as well as primary protease mutations absent from the ANRS list. Nevertheless, in the absence of large clinical studies on HIV-2 treatment failures, the evidence related to some mutations is based on small case series. Moreover the lists of mutations refer to the strain ROD from HIV-2 group A: it may skew the interpretation for group B, as some mutations are natural polymorphisms with no known effect on drug sensitivity in B strains. Besides the analysis of clinical samples related to virological failures, more studies depicting the phenotypic impact of mutations on isolates *in vitro* are warranted.

4.3 Indications

HIV-2 resistance tests are indicated in case of virological failure, i.e. presence of viral replication (detectable plasma viral load) under therapy. European guidelines for the clinical use of resistance tests recommend genotypic assays (Vandamme et al. 2011). As genetic barrier to resistance is low and therapeutic options limited, a resistance test should not be deferred once viral replication is detected.

In antiretroviral-naïve patients, HIV-2 resistance tests are not indicated in clinical practice. Even though some studies demonstrated the transmission of drug-resistant strains in West Africa and in Europe (Ruelle et al. 2007; Ruelle et al. 2008; Jallow et al. 2009), no data support the cost-effectiveness of such indication for HIV-2.

4.4 Tropism testing

No HIV-2 tropism assay suitable for clinical use has been currently developed. Besides the lack of phenotypic or genotypic assay, the guidelines on the clinical management of HIV-1 tropism (Vandekerckhove et al. 2011) do not apply to HIV-2 for the following reasons: the clinical outcome of CCR-5 antagonists containing regimen is unknown, few studies correlating the gp120 coding sequences and the phenotype are published and thus no genotypic interpretation rules exist (Dimonte et al. 2011), and the viral tropism extends to broader chemokine receptors for which the clinical relevance is controversial (Calado et al. 2010; Blaak et al. 2005).

5. Conclusions

Several challenges related to the diagnosis and the follow-up of HIV-2 infections need to be addressed:

- Although most HIV screening assays now detect antibodies directed against type 1 and 2 viruses, fourth generation tests have poorer sensitivity to HIV-2 antigens.
- The algorithms defining the number and which tests to use for HIV-2 diagnosis differ widely. This is related to varying prevalences between countries or continents, but is also related to the availability of tests, particularly nucleic acid tests. Those decision trees should be harmonised to ensure an accurate diagnosis: misidentification of HIV type has hazardous consequences for the clinical management.
- Reference standards for plasma viral load quantification will facilitate multi-centric collaborations, as a lack of consistency between assays has been observed. Although standards are now available for group A, quantification of other groups remains problematic. No commercial HIV-1 viral load platform is up to now applicable for HIV-2 in clinical settings.
- No clinically validated tropism assay is available, preventing the use of CCR-5 antagonists for HIV-2 treatment.
- The apparent reduced genetic barrier to antiretroviral resistance imposes a careful choice of drugs and a fine-tuning of genotypic interpretation rules.
- The majority of patients are long-term non-progressors or controllers; prediction of evolution and applying different follow-up patterns to controllers or progressors would rationalise the use of resources.

We have to keep in mind that the majority of HIV-2 patients live in countries where the diagnostics tools discussed here are not all available. More field evaluations in endemic regions, monitoring the impact of new laboratory tools, defining the best antiretroviral regimen, evaluating the prevalence of resistance and understanding better the pathways leading to treatment failure would supplement expert opinion rules with evidence-based data.

6. References

Amor, A., A. Simon, M. Salgado, B. Rodes, V. Soriano, and C. Toro. 2009. Lack of significant cross-reactivity for HIV-2 immunoblots in HIV-1-infected patients. *J Acquir Immune Defic Syndr* 50 (3):339-40.

Andersson, S., H. Norrgren, Z. da Silva, A. Biague, S. Bamba, S. Kwok, C. Christopherson, G. Biberfeld, and J. Albert. 2000. Plasma viral load in HIV-1 and HIV-2 singly and dually infected individuals in Guinea-Bissau, West Africa: significantly lower plasma virus set point in HIV-2 infection than in HIV-1 infection. *Arch Intern Med* 160 (21):3286-93.

Andries, K., H. Azijn, T. Thielemans, D. Ludovici, M. Kukla, J. Heeres, P. Janssen, B. De Corte, J. Vingerhoets, R. Pauwels, and M. P. de Bethune. 2004. TMC125, a novel next-generation nonnucleoside reverse transcriptase inhibitor active against nonnucleoside reverse transcriptase inhibitor-resistant human immunodeficiency virus type 1. *Antimicrob Agents Chemother* 48 (12):4680-6.

ANRS-AC11. *Genotype interpretation for HIV-2, www.hivfrenchresistance.org* 2011. Consulted 2011 Aug 18.

Armstrong-James, D., J. Stebbing, A. Scourfield, E. Smit, B. Ferns, D. Pillay, and M. Nelson. 2010. Clinical outcome in resistant HIV-2 infection treated with raltegravir and maraviroc. *Antiviral Res* 86 (2):224-6.

Barin, F., S. M'Boup, F. Denis, P. Kanki, J. S. Allan, T. H. Lee, and M. Essex. 1985. Serological evidence for virus related to simian T-lymphotropic retrovirus III in residents of west Africa. *Lancet* 2 (8469-70):1387-9.

Barin, F., F. Cazein, F. Lot, J. Pillonel, S. Brunet, D. Thierry, F. Damond, F. Brun-Vezinet, J. C. Desenclos, and C. Semaille. 2007. Prevalence of HIV-2 and HIV-1 group O infections among new HIV diagnoses in France: 2003-2006. *AIDS* 21 (17):2351-3.

Barre-Sinoussi, F., J. C. Chermann, F. Rey, M. T. Nugeyre, S. Chamaret, J. Gruest, C. Dauguet, C. Axler-Blin, F. Vezinet-Brun, C. Rouzioux, W. Rozenbaum, and L. Montagnier. 1983. Isolation of a T-lymphotropic retrovirus from a patient at risk for acquired immune deficiency syndrome (AIDS). *Science* 220 (4599):868-71.

Beelaert, G., and K. Fransen. 2010. Evaluation of a rapid and simple fourth-generation HIV screening assay for qualitative detection of HIV p24 antigen and/or antibodies to HIV-1 and HIV-2. *J Virol Methods* 168 (1-2):218-22.

Benard, A., A. van Sighem, A. Taieb, E. Valadas, J. Ruelle, V. Soriano, A. Calmy, C. Balotta, F. Damond, F. Brun-Vezinet, G. Chene, and S. Matheron. 2011. Immunovirological response to triple nucleotide reverse-transcriptase inhibitors and ritonavir-boosted protease inhibitors in treatment-naive HIV-2-infected patients: The ACHIEV2E Collaboration Study Group. *Clin Infect Dis* 52 (10):1257-66.

Bercoff, D. P., P. Triqueneaux, C. Lambert, A. A. Oumar, A. M. Ternes, S. Dao, P. Goubau, J. C. Schmit, and J. Ruelle. 2010. Polymorphisms of HIV-2 integrase and selection of resistance to raltegravir. *Retrovirology* 7:98.

Blaak, H., P. H. Boers, R. A. Gruters, H. Schuitemaker, M. E. van der Ende, and A. D. Osterhaus. 2005. CCR5, GPR15, and CXCR6 are major coreceptors of human immunodeficiency virus type 2 variants isolated from individuals with and without plasma viremia. *J Virol* 79 (3):1686-700.

Branson, B. M. 2010. The future of HIV testing. *J Acquir Immune Defic Syndr* 55 Suppl 2:S102-5.

Brower, E. T., U. M. Bacha, Y. Kawasaki, and E. Freire. 2008. Inhibition of HIV-2 protease by HIV-1 protease inhibitors in clinical use. *Chem Biol Drug Des* 71 (4):298-305.

Brun-Vezinet, F., M. A. Rey, C. Katlama, P. M. Girard, D. Roulot, P. Yeni, L. Lenoble, F. Clavel, M. Alizon, S. Gadelle, and et al. 1987. Lymphadenopathy-associated virus type 2 in AIDS and AIDS-related complex. Clinical and virological features in four patients. *Lancet* 1 (8525):128-32.

Burgard, M., C. Jasseron, S. Matheron, F. Damond, K. Hamrene, S. Blanche, A. Faye, C. Rouzioux, J. Warszawski, and L. Mandelbro. 2010. Mother-to-child transmission of HIV-2 infection from 1986 to 2007 in the ANRS French Perinatal Cohort EPF-CO1. *Clin Infect Dis* 51 (7):833-43.

Calado, M., P. Matoso, Q. Santos-Costa, M. Espirito-Santo, J. Machado, L. Rosado, F. Antunes, K. Mansinho, M. M. Lopes, F. Maltez, M. O. Santos-Ferreira, and J. M. Azevedo-Pereira. 2010. Coreceptor usage by HIV-1 and HIV-2 primary isolates: the relevance of CCR8 chemokine receptor as an alternative coreceptor. *Virology* 408 (2):174-82.

Campbell-Yesufu, O. T., and R. T. Gandhi. 2011. Update on human immunodeficiency virus (HIV)-2 infection. *Clin Infect Dis* 52 (6):780-7.

Centers for Disease Control [CDC] 2011. HIV-2 infection surveillance - United States, 1987-2009. *Morbidity and mortality weekly report (MMWR)* 60 (29):977-1008.

Chakrabarti, L., M. Guyader, M. Alizon, M. D. Daniel, R. C. Desrosiers, P. Tiollais, and P. Sonigo. 1987. Sequence of simian immunodeficiency virus from macaque and its relationship to other human and simian retroviruses. *Nature* 328 (6130):543-7.

Charpentier, C., B. Roquebert, O. Delelis, L. Larrouy, S. Matheron, R. Tubiana, M. Karmochkine, X. Duval, G. Chene, A. Storto, G. Collin, A. Benard, F. Damond, J. F. Mouscadet, F. Brun-Vezinet, and D. Descamps. 2011. Hot spots of integrase genotypic changes leading to HIV-2 resistance to raltegravir. *Antimicrob Agents Chemother* 55 (3):1293-5.

Ciccaglione, A. R., M. Miceli, G. Pisani, R. Bruni, P. Iudicone, A. Costantino, M. Equestre, E. Tritarelli, C. Marcantonio, P. Tataseo, M. C. Marazzi, S. Ceffa, G. Paturzo, A. M. Altan, M. M. San Lio, S. Mancinelli, M. Ciccozzi, A. Lo Presti, G. Rezza, and L. Palombi. 2010. Improving HIV-2 detection by a combination of serological and nucleic acid amplification test assays. *J Clin Microbiol* 48 (8):2902-8.

Clavel, F., D. Guetard, F. Brun-Vezinet, S. Chamaret, M. A. Rey, M. O. Santos-Ferreira, A. G. Laurent, C. Dauguet, C. Katlama, C. Rouzioux, and et al. 1986. Isolation of a new human retrovirus from West African patients with AIDS. *Science* 233 (4761):343-6.

Clavel, F., K. Mansinho, S. Chamaret, D. Guetard, V. Favier, J. Nina, M. O. Santos-Ferreira, J. L. Champalimaud, and L. Montagnier. 1987. Human immunodeficiency virus type 2 infection associated with AIDS in West Africa. *N Engl J Med* 316 (19):1180-5.

Colson, P., M. Henry, N. Tivoli, H. Gallais, J. A. Gastaut, J. Moreau, and C. Tamalet. 2005. Polymorphism and drug-selected mutations in the reverse transcriptase gene of HIV-2 from patients living in southeastern France. *J Med Virol* 75 (3):381-90.

da Silva, Z. J., I. Oliveira, A. Andersen, F. Dias, A. Rodrigues, B. Holmgren, S. Andersson, and P. Aaby. 2008. Changes in prevalence and incidence of HIV-1, HIV-2 and dual infections in urban areas of Bissau, Guinea-Bissau: is HIV-2 disappearing? *AIDS* 22 (10):1195-202.

Damond, F., C. Apetrei, D. L. Robertson, S. Souquiere, A. Lepretre, S. Matheron, J. C. Plantier, F. Brun-Vezinet, and F. Simon. 2001. Variability of human immunodeficiency virus type 2 (hiv-2) infecting patients living in france. *Virology* 280 (1):19-30.

Damond, F., D. Descamps, I. Farfara, J. N. Telles, S. Puyeo, P. Campa, A. Lepretre, S. Matheron, F. Brun-Vezinet, and F. Simon. 2001. Quantification of proviral load of human immunodeficiency virus type 2 subtypes A and B using real-time PCR. *J Clin Microbiol* 39 (12):4264-8.

Damond, F., M. Worobey, P. Campa, I. Farfara, G. Colin, S. Matheron, F. Brun-Vezinet, D. L. Robertson, and F. Simon. 2004. Identification of a highly divergent HIV type 2 and proposal for a change in HIV type 2 classification. *AIDS Res Hum Retroviruses* 20 (6):666-72.

Damond, F., G. Collin, S. Matheron, G. Peytavin, P. Campa, S. Delarue, A. Taieb, A. Benard, G. Chene, F. Brun-Vezinet, and D. Descamps. 2005. Letter. In vitro phenotypic susceptibility to nucleoside reverse transcriptase inhibitors of HIV-2 isolates with the Q151M mutation in the reverse transcriptase gene. *Antivir Ther* 10 (7):861-5.

Damond, F., S. Lariven, B. Roquebert, S. Males, G. Peytavin, G. Morau, D. Toledano, D. Descamps, F. Brun-Vezinet, and S. Matheron. 2008. Virological and immunological response to HAART regimen containing integrase inhibitors in HIV-2-infected patients. *AIDS* 22 (5):665-6.

Damond, F., A. Benard, J. Ruelle, A. Alabi, B. Kupfer, P. Gomes, B. Rodes, J. Albert, J. Boni, J. Garson, B. Ferns, S. Matheron, G. Chene, and F. Brun-Vezinet. 2008. Quality control assessment of human immunodeficiency virus type 2 (HIV-2) viral load quantification assays: results from an international collaboration on HIV-2 infection in 2006. *J Clin Microbiol* 46 (6):2088-91.

Damond, F., A. Benard, C. Balotta, J. Boni, M. Cotten, V. Duque, B. Ferns, J. Garson, P. Gomes, F. Goncalves, G. Gottlieb, B. Kupfer, J. Ruelle, B. Rodes, V. Soriano, M. Wainberg, A. Taieb, S. Matheron, G. Chene, and F. Brun-Vezinet. 2011. An international collaboration to standardize HIV-2 viral load assays: Results from the 2009 ACHIEV2E quality control study. *J Clin Microbiol.*

Desbois, D., B. Roquebert, G. Peytavin, F. Damond, G. Collin, A. Benard, P. Campa, S. Matheron, G. Chene, F. Brun-Vezinet, and D. Descamps. 2008. In vitro phenotypic susceptibility of human immunodeficiency virus type 2 clinical isolates to protease inhibitors. *Antimicrob Agents Chemother* 52 (4):1545-8.

Descamps, D., F. Damond, S. Matheron, G. Collin, P. Campa, S. Delarue, S. Pueyo, G. Chene, and F. Brun-Vezinet. 2004. High frequency of selection of K65R and Q151M mutations in HIV-2 infected patients receiving nucleoside reverse transcriptase inhibitors containing regimen. *J Med Virol* 74 (2):197-201.

Dimonte, S., V. Svicher, R. Salpini, F. Ceccherini-Silberstein, C. F. Perno, and M. Babakir-Mina. 2011. HIV-2 A-subtype gp125(C2-V3-C3) mutations and their association with CCR5 and CXCR4 tropism. *Arch Virol.*

Ferns, R. B., and J. A. Garson. 2006. Development and evaluation of a real-time RT-PCR assay for quantification of cell-free human immunodeficiency virus type 2 using a Brome Mosaic Virus internal control. *J Virol Methods* 135 (1):102-8.

Francisci, D., L. Martinelli, L. E. Weimer, M. Zazzi, M. Floridia, G. Masini, and F. Baldelli. 2011. HIV-2 infection, end-stage renal disease and protease inhibitor intolerance: which salvage regimen? *Clin Drug Investig* 31 (5):345-9.

Gao, F., L. Yue, D. L. Robertson, S. C. Hill, H. Hui, R. J. Biggar, A. E. Neequaye, T. M. Whelan, D. D. Ho, G. M. Shaw, and et al. 1994. Genetic diversity of human immunodeficiency virus type 2: evidence for distinct sequence subtypes with differences in virus biology. *J Virol* 68 (11):7433-47.

Gilleece, Y., D. R. Chadwick, J. Breuer, D. Hawkins, E. Smit, L. X. McCrae, D. Pillay, N. Smith, and J. Anderson. 2010. British HIV Association guidelines for antiretroviral treatment of HIV-2-positive individuals 2010. *HIV Med* 11 (10):611-9.

Gomes, P., A. Abecasis, M. Almeida, R. Camacho, and K. Mansinho. 2003. Transmission of HIV-2. *Lancet Infect Dis* 3 (11):683-4.

Gomes, P. , K. Van Laethem, A-M. Geretti, R. Camacho, and A-M. Vandamme. *Algorithm for the interpretation of genotypic HIV-2 resistance data, www.kuleuven.ac.be/rega/cew/links* 2009. Consulted 2011 Aug 18.

Gottlieb, G. S., P. S. Sow, S. E. Hawes, I. Ndoye, M. Redman, A. M. Coll-Seck, M. A. Faye-Niang, A. Diop, J. M. Kuypers, C. W. Critchlow, R. Respess, J. I. Mullins, and N. B. Kiviat. 2002. Equal plasma viral loads predict a similar rate of CD4+ T cell decline in human immunodeficiency virus (HIV) type 1- and HIV-2-infected individuals from Senegal, West Africa. *J Infect Dis* 185 (7):905-14.

Gottlieb, G. S., S. P. Eholie, J. N. Nkengasong, S. Jallow, S. Rowland-Jones, H. C. Whittle, and P. S. Sow. 2008. A call for randomized controlled trials of antiretroviral therapy for HIV-2 infection in West Africa. *AIDS* 22 (16):2069-72; discussion 2073-4.

Gottlieb, G. S., S. E. Hawes, N. B. Kiviat, and P. S. Sow. 2008. Differences in proviral DNA load between HIV-1-infected and HIV-2-infected patients. *AIDS* 22 (11):1379-80.

Gottlieb, G. S., R. A. Smith, N. M. Dia Badiane, S. Ba, S. E. Hawes, M. Toure, A. K. Starling, F. Traore, F. Sall, S. L. Cherne, J. Stern, K. G. Wong, P. Lu, M. Kim, D. N. Raugi, A. Lam, J. I. Mullins, and N. B. Kiviat. 2011. HIV-2 Integrase Variation in Integrase Inhibitor-Naive Adults in Senegal, West Africa. *PLoS One* 6 (7):e22204.

Gueudin, M., F. Damond, J. Braun, A. Taieb, V. Lemee, J. C. Plantier, G. Chene, S. Matheron, F. Brun-Vezinet, and F. Simon. 2008. Differences in proviral DNA load between HIV-1- and HIV-2-infected patients. *AIDS* 22 (2):211-5.

Hirsch, V. M., R. A. Olmsted, M. Murphey-Corb, R. H. Purcell, and P. R. Johnson. 1989. An African primate lentivirus (SIVsm) closely related to HIV-2. *Nature* 339 (6223):389-92.

Huet, T., R. Cheynier, A. Meyerhans, G. Roelants, and S. Wain-Hobson. 1990. Genetic organization of a chimpanzee lentivirus related to HIV-1. *Nature* 345 (6273):356-9.

Ibe, S., Y. Yokomaku, T. Shiino, R. Tanaka, J. Hattori, S. Fujisaki, Y. Iwatani, N. Mamiya, M. Utsumi, S. Kato, M. Hamaguchi, and W. Sugiura. 2010. HIV-2 CRF01_AB: first circulating recombinant form of HIV-2. *J Acquir Immune Defic Syndr* 54 (3):241-7.

Jaffar, S., A. D. Grant, J. Whitworth, P. G. Smith, and H. Whittle. 2004. The natural history of HIV-1 and HIV-2 infections in adults in Africa: a literature review. *Bull World Health Organ* 82 (6):462-9.

Jallow, S., T. Vincent, A. Leligdowicz, T. De Silva, C. Van Tienen, A. Alabi, R. Sarge-Njie, P. Aaby, T. Corrah, H. Whittle, A. Jaye, G. Vanham, S. Rowland-Jones, and W. Janssens. 2009. Presence of a multidrug-resistance mutation in an HIV-2 variant

infecting a treatment-naive individual in Caio, Guinea Bissau. *Clin Infect Dis* 48 (12):1790-3.
Kania, D., P. Fao, D. Valea, C. Gouem, T. Kagone, H. Hien, P. Somda, P. Ouedraogo, A. Drabo, S. Gampini, N. Meda, S. Diagbouga, P. Van de Perre, and F. Rouet. 2010. Low prevalence rate of indeterminate serological human immunodeficiency virus results among pregnant women from Burkina Faso, West Africa. *J Clin Microbiol* 48 (4):1333-6.
Kanki, P. J. 1991. Biologic features of HIV-2. An update. *AIDS Clin Rev*:17-38.
Laurent, C., C. Kouanfack, G. Laborde-Balen, A. F. Aghokeng, J. B. Mbougua, S. Boyer, M. P. Carrieri, J. M. Mben, M. Dontsop, S. Kaze, N. Molinari, A. Bourgeois, E. Mpoudi-Ngole, B. Spire, S. Koulla-Shiro, and E. Delaporte. 2011. Monitoring of HIV viral loads, CD4 cell counts, and clinical assessments versus clinical monitoring alone for antiretroviral therapy in rural district hospitals in Cameroon (Stratall ANRS 12110/ESTHER): a randomised non-inferiority trial. *Lancet Infect Dis* doi:10.1016/S1473-3099(11)70168-2
Leligdowicz, A., and S. Rowland-Jones. 2008. Tenets of protection from progression to AIDS: lessons from the immune responses to HIV-2 infection. *Expert Rev Vaccines* 7 (3):319-31.
Leligdowicz, A., C. Onyango, L. M. Yindom, Y. Peng, M. Cotten, A. Jaye, A. McMichael, H. Whittle, T. Dong, and S. Rowland-Jones. 2010. Highly avid, oligoclonal, early-differentiated antigen-specific CD8+ T cells in chronic HIV-2 infection. *Eur J Immunol* 40 (7):1963-72.
Lemey, P., O. G. Pybus, B. Wang, N. K. Saksena, M. Salemi, and A. M. Vandamme. 2003. Tracing the origin and history of the HIV-2 epidemic. *Proc Natl Acad Sci U S A* 100 (11):6588-92.
Letvin, N. L., M. D. Daniel, P. K. Sehgal, R. C. Desrosiers, R. D. Hunt, L. M. Waldron, J. J. MacKey, D. K. Schmidt, L. V. Chalifoux, and N. W. King. 1985. Induction of AIDS-like disease in macaque monkeys with T-cell tropic retrovirus STLV-III. *Science* 230 (4721):71-3.
Martinez-Steele, E., A. A. Awasana, T. Corrah, S. Sabally, M. van der Sande, A. Jaye, T. Togun, R. Sarge-Njie, S. J. McConkey, H. Whittle, and M. F. Schim van der Loeff. 2007. Is HIV-2- induced AIDS different from HIV-1-associated AIDS? Data from a West African clinic. *AIDS* 21 (3):317-24.
McKellar, M. S., P. Jongthavorn, and H. Khanlou. 2008. False-positivity of HIV-2 immunoblots in a cohort of elite suppressors infected with HIV-1. *J Acquir Immune Defic Syndr* 47 (5):644.
Naucler, A., P. A. Andreasson, C. M. Costa, R. Thorstensson, and G. Biberfeld. 1989. HIV-2-associated AIDS and HIV-2 seroprevalence in Bissau, Guinea-Bissau. *J Acquir Immune Defic Syndr* 2 (1):88-93.
Ntemgwa, M. L., T. d'Aquin Toni, B. G. Brenner, R. J. Camacho, and M. A. Wainberg. 2009. Antiretroviral drug resistance in human immunodeficiency virus type 2. *Antimicrob Agents Chemother* 53 (9):3611-9.
O'Donovan, D., K. Ariyoshi, P. Milligan, M. Ota, L. Yamuah, R. Sarge-Njie, and H. Whittle. 2000. Maternal plasma viral RNA levels determine marked differences in mother-to-child transmission rates of HIV-1 and HIV-2 in The Gambia. MRC/Gambia

Government/University College London Medical School working group on mother-child transmission of HIV. *AIDS* 14 (4):441-8.

Padua, E., C. Almeida, B. Nunes, H. Cortes Martins, J. Castela, C. Neves, and M. T. Paixao. 2009. Assessment of mother-to-child HIV-1 and HIV-2 transmission: an AIDS reference laboratory collaborative study. *HIV Med* 10 (3):182-90.

Peterson, K., S. Jallow, S. L. Rowland-Jones, and T. I. de Silva. 2011. Antiretroviral Therapy for HIV-2 Infection: Recommendations for Management in Low-Resource Settings. *AIDS Res Treat* 2011:463704.

Poljak, M., E. Smit, and J. Ross. 2009. 2008 European Guideline on HIV testing. *Int J STD AIDS* 20 (2):77-83.

Poulsen, A. G., P. Aaby, A. Gottschau, B. B. Kvinesdal, F. Dias, K. Molbak, and E. Lauritzen. 1993. HIV-2 infection in Bissau, West Africa, 1987-1989: incidence, prevalences, and routes of transmission. *J Acquir Immune Defic Syndr* 6 (8):941-8.

Poulsen, A. G., P. Aaby, H. Jensen, and F. Dias. 2000. Risk factors for HIV-2 seropositivity among older people in Guinea-Bissau. A search for the early history of HIV-2 infection. *Scand J Infect Dis* 32 (2):169-75.

Poveda, E., B. Rodes, C. Toro, and V. Soriano. 2004. Are fusion inhibitors active against all HIV variants? *AIDS Res Hum Retroviruses* 20 (3):347-8.

Qiu, M., X. Liu, Y. Jiang, J. N. Nkengasong, W. Xing, L. Pei, and B. S. Parekh. 2009. Current HIV-2 diagnostic strategy overestimates HIV-2 prevalence in China. *J Med Virol* 81 (5):790-7.

Rodes, B., J. Sheldon, C. Toro, L. Cuevas, E. Perez-Pastrana, I. Herrera, and V. Soriano. 2007. Quantitative detection of plasma human immunodeficiency virus type 2 subtype A RNA by the Nuclisens EasyQ Assay (version 1.1). *J Clin Microbiol* 45 (1):88-92.

Rodes, B., J. Sheldon, C. Toro, V. Jimenez, M. A. Alvarez, and V. Soriano. 2006. Susceptibility to protease inhibitors in HIV-2 primary isolates from patients failing antiretroviral therapy. *J Antimicrob Chemother* 57 (4):709-13.

Roquebert, B., F. Damond, G. Collin, S. Matheron, G. Peytavin, A. Benard, P. Campa, G. Chene, F. Brun-Vezinet, and D. Descamps. 2008. HIV-2 integrase gene polymorphism and phenotypic susceptibility of HIV-2 clinical isolates to the integrase inhibitors raltegravir and elvitegravir in vitro. *J Antimicrob Chemother* 62 (5):914-20.

Rowland-Jones, S. L., and H. C. Whittle. 2007. Out of Africa: what can we learn from HIV-2 about protective immunity to HIV-1? *Nat Immunol* 8 (4):329-31.

Ruelle, J., B. K. Mukadi, M. Schutten, and P. Goubau. 2004. Quantitative real-time PCR on Lightcycler for the detection of human immunodeficiency virus type 2 (HIV-2). *J Virol Methods* 117 (1):67-74.

Ruelle, J., M. Sanou, H. F. Liu, A. T. Vandenbroucke, A. Duquenne, and P. Goubau. 2007. Genetic polymorphisms and resistance mutations of HIV type 2 in antiretroviral-naive patients in Burkina Faso. *AIDS Res Hum Retroviruses* 23 (8):955-64.

Ruelle, J., F. Roman, A. T. Vandenbroucke, C. Lambert, K. Fransen, F. Echahidi, D. Pierard, C. Verhofstede, K. Van Laethem, M. L. Delforge, D. Vaira, J. C. Schmit, and P. Goubau. 2008. Transmitted drug resistance, selection of resistance mutations and moderate antiretroviral efficacy in HIV-2: analysis of the HIV-2 Belgium and Luxembourg database. *BMC Infect Dis* 8:21.

Sangare, K. A., I. M. Coulibaly, and A. Ehouman. 1998. [Seroprevalence of HIV among pregnant women in the ten regions of the Ivory Coast]. *Sante* 8 (3):193-8.

Schim van der Loeff, M. F., S. Jaffar, A. A. Aveika, S. Sabally, T. Corrah, E. Harding, A. Alabi, A. Bayang, K. Ariyoshi, and H. C. Whittle. 2002. Mortality of HIV-1, HIV-2 and HIV-1/HIV-2 dually infected patients in a clinic-based cohort in The Gambia. *AIDS* 16 (13):1775-83.

Schutten, M., B. van den Hoogen, M. E. van der Ende, R. A. Gruters, A. D. Osterhaus, and H. G. Niesters. 2000. Development of a real-time quantitative RT-PCR for the detection of HIV-2 RNA in plasma. *J Virol Methods* 88 (1):81-7.

Schutten, M. 2006. Resistance assays. In *Antiretroviral resistance in clinical practice*, edited by A.-M. Geretti. London: Mediscript.

Sharp, P. M., E. Bailes, R. R. Chaudhuri, C. M. Rodenburg, M. O. Santiago, and B. H. Hahn. 2001. The origins of acquired immune deficiency syndrome viruses: where and when? *Philos Trans R Soc Lond B Biol Sci* 356 (1410):867-76.

Smith, R. A., D. J. Anderson, C. L. Pyrak, B. D. Preston, and G. S. Gottlieb. 2009. Antiretroviral drug resistance in HIV-2: three amino acid changes are sufficient for classwide nucleoside analogue resistance. *J Infect Dis* 199 (9):1323-6.

Talha, S. M., T. Salminen, S. Swaminathan, T. Soukka, K. Pettersson, and N. Khanna. 2011. A highly sensitive and specific time resolved fluorometric bridge assay for antibodies to HIV-1 and -2. *J Virol Methods* 173 (1):24-30.

Thiébaut, R., S. Matheron, A. Taieb, F. Brun-Vezinet, G. Chene, and B. Autran. 2011. Long-term nonprogressors and elite controllers in the ANRS CO5 HIV-2 cohort. *AIDS* 25 (6):865-7.

Torian, L. V., J. J. Eavey, A. P. Punsalang, R. E. Pirillo, L. A. Forgione, S. A. Kent, and W. R. Oleszko. 2010. HIV type 2 in New York City, 2000-2008. *Clin Infect Dis* 51 (11):1334-42.

Valadas, E., L. Franca, S. Sousa, and F. Antunes. 2009. 20 years of HIV-2 infection in Portugal: trends and changes in epidemiology. *Clin Infect Dis* 48 (8):1166-7.

van Tienen, C., M. S. van der Loeff, S. M. Zaman, T. Vincent, R. Sarge-Njie, I. Peterson, A. Leligdowicz, A. Jaye, S. Rowland-Jones, P. Aaby, and H. Whittle. 2010. Two distinct epidemics: the rise of HIV-1 and decline of HIV-2 infection between 1990 and 2007 in rural Guinea-Bissau. *J Acquir Immune Defic Syndr* 53 (5):640-7.

Vandamme, A. M., R. J. Camacho, F. Ceccherini-Silberstein, A. de Luca, L. Palmisano, D. Paraskevis, R. Paredes, M. Poljak, J. C. Schmit, V. Soriano, H. Walter, and A. Sonnerborg. 2011. European recommendations for the clinical use of HIV drug resistance testing: 2011 update. *AIDS Rev* 13 (2):77-108.

Vandekerckhove, L. P., A. M. Wensing, R. Kaiser, F. Brun-Vezinet, B. Clotet, A. De Luca, S. Dressler, F. Garcia, A. M. Geretti, T. Klimkait, K. Korn, B. Masquelier, C. F. Perno, J. M. Schapiro, V. Soriano, A. Sonnerborg, A. M. Vandamme, C. Verhofstede, H. Walter, M. Zazzi, and C. A. Boucher. 2011. European guidelines on the clinical management of HIV-1 tropism testing. *Lancet Infect Dis* 11 (5):394-407.

Winters, B., J. Montaner, P. R. Harrigan, B. Gazzard, A. Pozniak, M. D. Miller, S. Emery, F. van Leth, P. Robinson, J. D. Baxter, M. Perez-Elias, D. Castor, S. Hammer, A. Rinehart, H. Vermeiren, E. Van Craenenbroeck, and L. Bacheler. 2008. Determination of clinically relevant cutoffs for HIV-1 phenotypic resistance estimates through a combined analysis of clinical trial and cohort data. *J Acquir Immune Defic Syndr* 48 (1):26-34.

Witvrouw, M., C. Pannecouque, W. M. Switzer, T. M. Folks, E. De Clercq, and W. Heneine. 2004. Susceptibility of HIV-2, SIV and SHIV to various anti-HIV-1 compounds: implications for treatment and postexposure prophylaxis. *Antivir Ther* 9 (1):57-65.

Yamaguchi, J., A. Vallari, N. Ndembi, R. Coffey, C. Ngansop, D. Mbanya, L. Kaptue, L. G. Gurtler, S. G. Devare, and C. A. Brennan. 2008. HIV type 2 intergroup recombinant identified in Cameroon. *AIDS Res Hum Retroviruses* 24 (1):86-91.

3

Personal Computer, Mobile Phone and Internet Technologies to Increase HIV Testing and Prevention

Sonia A. Alemagno and Deric R. Kenne
Kent State University,
College of Public Health
United States

1. Introduction

Globally, since the AIDS epidemic began, nearly 60 million individuals have contracted HIV with 25 million having died from causes related to the infection (World Health Organization [WHO], 2009). In 2009, it was estimated that 33.4 million people world-wide were living with HIV (WHO, 2009). The Centers for Disease Control and Prevention (CDC) estimates that over one million individuals in the United States are living with HIV, and since the 1990s, the annual rate of individuals newly infected with HIV has remained relatively stable at about 56, 300 (CDC, 2010).

While the number of individuals reporting ever having been tested for HIV has been increasing steadily over time (Kaiser Family Foundation, 2006), a fifth (21%) of the HIV-infected population is unaware they are infected. This is an alarming statistic that continues to hamper efforts to substantially reduce the spread of the disease and improve the health of the public (CDC, 2010). Further, according to the CDC, among individuals appearing to a CDC-funded HIV-testing site in 2000, only 31% of those who tested positive for HIV ever returned to receive the results of the test (CDC, 2003).

Advances in medicine have proven effective in improving the quality of life of those who are HIV-positive. However, these improvements are more fully realized when HIV-positive status is identified early on. Early identification of HIV-positive status can be important in reducing morbidity and mortality (CDC, 2006), and studies have shown that individuals who are aware that they are HIV-positive will modify their behavior in an effort to prevent transmission of the virus (Marks et al., 2005).

The public health benefits of increased rates of HIV testing and awareness of HIV-positive status are clear. Consequently, strategies to increase HIV-testing, awareness of positive status, and motivation to obtain medical care are important in the effort to reduce the negative impact of HIV/AIDS. Today's technologies have the potential to substantially impact the AIDS epidemic by providing innovative and cost-effective means by which to reach more individuals and increase HIV-testing rates, awareness and motivation to change health behavior related to HIV/AIDS.

Researchers and clinicians working to influence and promote health behavior have only just begun to scratch the surface with regard to the uses of technologies in prevention and intervention programs. Examples that utilize technology to influence and promote health behavior include, but are not limited to, sending text messages to remind individuals of health care appointments, creating websites that provide specific health-related information and motivate individuals to seek health care services, and using tablet PCs or other mobile technologies to reach hidden populations and to administer assessments and interventions electronically. The potential for integrating and utilizing technology into health programs to influence and promote behavior is great and will continue to grow at a rapid pace. It is possible that as society continues to become more reliant on such technologies, health programs not utilizing or incorporating technologies will become less effective in comparison to technology-based health programs.

2. Advantages to using technology with HIV-positive and at-risk populations

The availability of, and advances in, personal computers, mobile phones and the Internet have grown exponentially over the last several years and growth continues at a staggering pace. As such, the use of these technologies is far reaching—impacting society in multiple ways. While the use of technology is pervasive in many ways, its application and potential benefit in raising awareness of and changing health behavior is much less pervasive, and thus potentially severely underutilized. To understand how technologies such as mobile phones, computers and the Internet can potentially positively impact the fight against HIV/AIDS, a general overview of the advantages of using or incorporating technology into programs created to change health behavior follows.

The use of technology to raise awareness of health concerns such as HIV-positive status and facilitate health behavior change is a relatively new and substantially understudied area. Given the apparent advantages to utilizing and incorporating technologies to impact the health outcomes of the public, including underserved populations, this line of research is likely to grow significantly over the next several years. The use and integration of technologies to influence and promote health behavior has several potential advantages (c.f., Bull, 2011). Below we reiterate and expand on the advantages of using technologies to influence and promote health as originally described by Bull (2011).

Reach. Perhaps the most significant and fundamental contribution technologies such as computers, mobile phones and the Internet have on promoting and changing health behavior is that of reach. Bull (2011) argues that the Internet offers an unprecedented opportunity to reach untold numbers of individuals. Likewise, the growing use and affordability of portable computers and mobile phones extends opportunities to connect with greater numbers of individuals. As a result, the effort to positively influence the health of the public can expand past traditional means of contact and interaction, thus reaching and impacting far more individuals than was previously thought possible. The use of the Internet, computers and mobile phones to promote and change health behavior has the potential to overcome many of the barriers that limit or preclude access to health programs (e.g., transportation and/or child care, inflexible work schedules of patients) (see, for example, DeLeon, Wakefield, & Hagglund, 2003; Nordal, Copans, & Stamm, 2003; Organista, Munoz, & Gonzalez, 1994; Stamm, 2003). This is especially true for women and minority individuals who are preferentially impacted by these barriers (Connell, Sanders, &

Markie-Dadds, 1997; National Institute of Mental Health, 2003; US Census Bureau, 2002; Weismann & Jensen, 2002). Highlighting the need to discover ways to overcome barriers, authors have noted that while a health program may be found efficacious, it may not necessarily have a substantial impact if it cannot reach the target population and engage that population over time for sustained effects (see Thyrian & Ulrich, 2007; Glasgow, Klesges, Dzewaltowski, Estabrooks, & Vogt, 2006; Klesges, Estabrooks, Dzewaltowski, Bull, & Glasgow, 2007).

Tailored Content. Technology can allow for health programs and interventions to be tailored to address patient factors (e.g., language barriers, low self-efficacy) and cushion provider bias (e.g. cognitive bias) and real-world system constraints (e.g., second/third-shift workers). Disadvantaged individuals tend to be more severely impacted by these factors and recent studies have shown that interactive multimedia computer programs can lessen these impacts (Jerant, Sohler, Fiscella, Franks, & Franks, 2010). Studies also indicate that information tailored to an individual becomes more relevant to the individual and thus is more likely to be read, comprehended and stored (Kreuter, Farrell, Olevitch, & Brennan, 2000; Stretcher, 1999). For instance, a computer-based health program designed to educate about the dangers of drug use can be programmed to discuss only issues related to drugs with which the respondent has indicated experience. A video-based health program would play through the dangers of all drugs, regardless of a drug's relevance to the respondent. As a result, respondents may become uninterested in the health program and fatigued by it because of what may be considered irrelevant information.

Feasibility. The use of technology in health programs and interventions can make the adoption, implementation and utilization of programs more feasible for community agencies. Glasgow, Lichtenstein, and Marcus (2003) argue that in order to reach some populations and have an impact on those populations, health programs must be made easy for community agencies to adopt, implement and utilize. Preliminary studies utilizing technology to promote health have shown that technology integration has promising potential to provide the means by which community agencies can easily implement and utilize proven health programs (Leeman-Castillo, Beaty, Raghunath, Steiner, & Bull, 2010; Cullen & Thompson, 2008; Skinner, Rivette, & Bloomberg, 2007). In short, utilizing a computer-based health program or intervention is often easier to implement and less expensive than hiring and training staff to deliver the same intervention.

Cost-Effectiveness. Technologies have the potential to lower costs associated with implementing and sustaining health programs and interventions. For example, the portability of computers, mobile phones and the Internet increases reach and reduces reliance on physical locations that require maintenance and which are often limited by size (see, for example, Booth, Nowson, & Matters, 2008; Brendryen & Kraft, 2008; Rainie, Horrigan, Wellman, & Boase, 2006). Home care programs can use camera phones to monitor patient wounds (estimated at 25% of home health admissions), thereby increasing the appropriate use of specialist services and decreasing associated costs (Sugrue & Riggs, 2005). Video phones used with patients receiving palliative care and antenatal home care have been shown to decrease isolation, save travel time and allow care team members to meet at a distance (Miyazaki, Stuart, Liu, Tell, & Stewart, 2003).

Standardization. Using technologies such as the Internet, mobile phones and computers, health programs can more readily standardize the content and delivery of the program.

Standardization helps ensure that each participant in the health program or intervention gets the content of the program exactly as it was intended. Further, standardization reduces variability, especially with regard to interactions with counselors or other content deliverers, and can substantially increase adherence to program curricula.

Interactive. Health programs can be technologically-enhanced to allow for a higher degree of interactivity than past means of health information delivery, such as video recordings and simple text-based or audio-assisted computer applications. For example, computers, mobile phones and the Internet can deliver health program content in multiple formats, including video-game formats. Similarly, health programs can be designed to mimic real-life interactivity with a counselor or other health care professional through the use of human simulation and artificial intelligence programs. Further, given that younger individuals are substantially more tech-savvy and reliant on technology, these individuals may, in fact, prefer interacting through computers, mobile phones and the Internet.

Anonymity & Confidentiality. While some caveats apply, technologies more readily offer anonymity to recipients of health programs and interventions. For example, through the use of a computer or mobile phone with Internet access, individuals can access and receive health program information and interventions without ever being personally identified. Likewise, technologies can store respondent information confidentially by generating unique identification codes or using biometric identification such as fingerprints, which can link several sources of data without identifying respondents.

Autonomy. Using technologies such as mobile phones, computers and the Internet, individuals can move through programs and interventions at their own pace. Further, individuals can be afforded the flexibility of accessing programs and interventions at times that are most convenient to them. For example, individuals who have work schedules that vary from week to week may not be able to readily access treatment or intervention services or may have trouble keeping appointments can benefit from the flexibility of accessing programs and services online at times and from locations convenient to their schedule.

Portability. Increasingly, over the past several years technologies have become more portable. Likewise, Internet access, especially free access, has become increasingly more common. Together, portability and Internet access allow individuals to easily access online content. Advances in mobile phone technologies (e.g., "smartphones") allow for the potential to create health prevention and intervention programs using software programs ("Apps") that can be downloaded to a smartphone and accessed anytime and anywhere, often without needing access to the Internet.

Storage & Backup. Technologies provide relatively easy and inexpensive storage and backup of information and can range from basic hard-drives or portable drives (e.g., flash drive, external hard drive) to more sophisticated devices such as secured networked drives with automatic and redundant backup. Further, electronic storage and backup can safeguard against information loss due to theft or disaster. For example, automatic backup and storage to a remote off-site location can protect information that might otherwise be destroyed in an on-site fire or other similar disaster.

The aforementioned discussion of the use of technology to influence and promote health behavior, including HIV-related testing and behavior, highlights the many potential advantages of using technology. Perhaps most importantly, technologies afford community

Advantage	Example
Reach	• Access to the Internet through free Wi-Fi is increasing. • Mobile phones ("smartphones") that can access the Internet have become more affordable. • Smart phones are able to run computer programs ("Apps"). • Internet-, computer- and mobile phone-delivered programs have the potential to always be on—allowing access at any time.
Tailored Content	• Programs can be tailored to the individual characteristics of the participant (e.g., an African-American female counselor can appear in a video for an African-American female client). • Content can be tailored based on the responses of the participant.
Feasibility	• Programs or interventions can be implemented with little or no training of staff, thus reducing potential costs to the agency. • An agency with limited staff may be able to provide additional services by utilizing technologies.
Cost-Effective	• Technologies can be utilized in place of more expensive program staff. • Technologies can reduce costs of training staff to conduct programming that can be done by a computer or other technology. • Technologies can be utilized off-site and have the ability to reach more individuals.
Standardization	• Content can be delivered exactly the same way each time. • Technologies can increase program fidelity. • Technologies can reduce the variability associated with individual differences of those delivering program content.
Interactive	• Technologies allow for interaction with computers, which may be more comforting for some participants, especially younger participants. • Content can be delivered using an approach that utilizes multiple forms of media (e.g., video, audio, games).
Anonymity & Confidentiality	• Participants can provide information or interact with a program anonymously through the Internet. • Participants can provide information or interact with programs on-site without revealing personally identifying information. • Technologies reduce the risk of breach of confidentiality because there are no hardcopy or paper formats of participant information.
Autonomy	• Participants can proceed through curricula or programming at their own pace without significant disruption to other participants or program staff.
Portability	• Technologies can be mobile and thus can remain in contact with the participant—providing continuous monitoring, support or communication.
Storage & Backup	• Participant information can be safely stored and backed-up to safeguard against theft or disaster.

Table 1. Examples of each potential advantage of using technologies to promote health.

agencies that serve at-risk HIV populations more options in which to provide services within limited and often shrinking operating budgets. For instance, as a result of federal and state cuts in funding for services, including services for minority populations (Zeanah, Stafford, & Zeanah, 2005), there have been calls to support the adoption of interventions that can be delivered in nontraditional and innovative ways that overcome traditional barriers to treatment provision and utilization (Hollon et al., 2002; National Institute of Mental Health, 2003).

Affordability of technology makes it increasingly possible for community agencies even in the poorest of neighborhoods, to utilize technology and technology-based services. As a result, technologies or technology-enhanced services can be more readily adopted, implemented and maintained allowing greater penetration into populations that are at risk for HIV. Additionally, the use of technology and technology-enhanced services allows agencies to expand evidence-based practices (EBPs) with minimal strain to limited staff and resources that are already stretched thin in many community agencies. Thus, technologies and technology-enhanced services can provide feasible real-world and evidence-based solutions that can reach even the most remote and underserved populations of individuals at risk for or living with HIV/AIDS.

3. Emerging literature

The emerging body of literature on computer-based interventions (including delivery via local computer or Internet, smart phone and social media) as applied to HIV testing, awareness and prevention shows great promise. Researchers point out that technological applications are especially important because significant investments have been made in the development of HIV prevention and behavioral interventions; however, there remain barriers to widespread use. These barriers include, but are not limited to, the cost of delivery (that is, requiring a human facilitator), maintenance to fidelity of interventions and distribution to remote or rural areas.

Noar (2011) presents a review of computer technology-based interventions in HIV prevention including interventions that are group-targeted, individually tailored and apply interactive video. The author presents a series of intriguing research questions regarding the use of technologies along the lines of reach (who are the appropriate audiences?), efficacy (what kinds of effects are possible?), adoption (who uses the technology?), implementation (what are the process issues?) and maintenance (how can the use of technology be sustained over time?). This work provides a framework for analyzing the newly emerging studies on the use of technology to promote HIV prevention.

Seeking health information online has become routine for most Americans. As such, it is no surprise that the Internet has been shown to be a source of sexual health information. Lesbian, gay, bisexual and transgender (LGBT) youth report that they use the Internet to seek sexual health information, particularly to avoid the stigma associated with asking questions of health care providers (Magee, Bigelow, DeHann, & Mustanski, 2011). Hightow-Weidman et. al (2011) developed a theory-based HIV/STI website for young, Black men who have sex with men (MSM) based on the Institute of Medicine's integrated model of behavior change and with input from young Black MSM focus group participants. Their interactive web site design uses live chats, quizzes, personalized health and "hook up/sex" journals. Clients reported high satisfaction with the approach, particularly due to its high cultural relevance. Therefore, websites present the opportunity to tailor health information in a way that can be continuously updated, as opposed to brochures in print.

Most studies of the Internet and HIV prevention have focused on gay, bisexual, and MSM who seek sexual partners online. These interventions have sought to promote HIV testing. A community-based participatory research (CBPR) partnership developed and piloted *CyBER/testing,* an intervention using Internet chat rooms set up to promote HIV testing among MSM "chatters" (MSM who use the chat room). The intervention showed a significant increase in self-reported testing for the chatters overall (Rhodes, et. al, 2011). This result was also supported by a study promoting testing via an online community for high-risk clients in North Carolina (Feldacker, et. al, 2010). Holt et. al (2011) in Australia found that the Internet is an important way to promote HIV testing among MSM. In particular, this study found that Internet social networks present the opportunity to engage never-tested clients in chat rooms which leads to increased motivation for testing. Bowen et. al (2008) examined the use of the Internet to conduct HIV prevention outreach to rural MSM. Overall, their findings suggest that web-based interventions may make rural outreach more feasible.

Clearly, Internet and social networking holds promise for reaching adolescent populations, given the documented high use of technology among this age group. Bull et. al (2007) developed a theoretically-based online HIV/STD and pregnancy prevention intervention aimed at 15-25 year old participants. The youth in this study felt that role model-delivered messages about HIV/STD and pregnancy risk, attitudes about condoms, norms and self-efficacy for negotiation would have a high impact. The youth preferred highly interactive websites such as chat rooms and message boards. The participants also felt that effective websites would give facts and real stories; however, they felt that reading should be short and to the point.

An interesting target population is that of homeless adolescents. A recent study (Young and Rice, 2011) found that in a sample of 201 homeless youth in Los Angeles, 79% reported using MySpace and/or Facebook almost every week. The adolescents used the Internet sites to communicate with others about drinking, drugs, parties, sex, being homeless and school experiences. The authors found that online social networks can be associated with both potential increases and potential decreases in HIV/STD risk among homeless youth. As an example of potential increases in HIV/STD risk, some homeless youth reported that they used social network sites to sell sex. Overall, however, online social network use was associated with increased knowledge and HIV/STD prevention behaviors among homeless youth. The authors conclude that homeless youth need more access to the Internet, since access may facilitate contact with family and home-based peers. This contact was found to be associated with decreased risk and increased testing. However, the authors caution that online environments need to be carefully monitored to prevent youth from soliciting sex online.

Using the Internet to reach high-risk individuals is a strategy being used in HIV prevention globally. Blas et. al (2007) used an Internet intervention in Peru to access high risk MSM. In this context, the authors describe how Peruvian MSM are shifting from physical to virtual places, not only to look for sexual partners but also to look for HIV-related health information. The study concluded that attracting high-risk MSM not tested for HIV to an intervention may be feasible by on-line recruitment.

Brief computerized interventions to reduce risk and increase HIV testing have been found to be effective. Alemagno et. al (2009) developed and implemented a computerized, self-administered HIV/STD risk screen using the "brief negotiation interviewing" (BNI) approach. Participants were able to answer a set of risk questions via computer, receive immediate risk feedback and work through a plan to increase motivation for testing. The participants in the computerized BNI intervention group were more likely to obtain an HIV test by the 3-month follow-up interview as compared to the controls. Grimley and Hook (2009) also found that a 15-minute interactive, computerized condom use intervention increased condom use. The intervention was conducted in a clinical setting and self-administered by the participants. The authors concluded that the intervention held considerable promise in that there was no additional burden on clinicians or staff.

Another promising technology for HIV prevention is the use of mobile phones. A recent study finds that riskier youth (in terms of HIV/STI risk behavior) are online and using cell phones frequently (Whiteley et. al, 2011). This study of over 1,500 African American adolescents found that over 90% of adolescents used their cell phones every day and 60% used social networking sites. The authors conclude that mobile phone interventions may be promising to reducing risks by providing health information.

Text messaging is an application that is emerging to reach target populations. A pilot program aimed at young Black men using a 12-week text message program found that the intervention group showed a trend toward increased monogamy at follow-up compared to controls (Juzang, Fortune, Black, Wright, & Bull, 2011). The intervention group also had higher awareness of sexual health compared to the controls. Another study found that young persons have positive attitudes toward text messages as appointment or medication reminders or for health information related to HIV (Person, Blain, Jiang, Rasmussen, & Stout, 2011). Receiving a text message was perceived as more acceptable than having to answer the phone. A message could be saved for viewing at a later time. One drawback of using text messages is that target populations must have sufficient literacy and there is the obvious cost associated with a mobile phone with text capabilities. This study also points out that less frequent, targeted reminders are most acceptable so the frequency is an important consideration.

4. Cautions in using technologies

While the use of technologies such as computers, mobile phones and the Internet show significant promise, careful consideration should be given to address any potential concerns. Below we discuss several potential issues that could arise when utilizing technologies in health-promoting programs for populations living with or at risk for HIV/AIDS. As more research emerges on the topic of technology-based health promotion, so should solutions to these potential issues.

Literacy. Even though it is possible to program computers to read text to participants, the use of health education websites or the use of health messages sent by text message requires participants to have the ability to read and understand the content. Few studies have examined the impact of literacy on mobile device use.

Confidentiality. There are confidentiality concerns regarding information that is disclosed on Internet sites and mobile devices, including risks related to self-disclosure and risks related to unintended persons viewing information transmitted to mobile devices. While providers may feel assured that they are transmitting information to the correct person based on a mobile number, there is no control over who is reading the information once delivered to the device. Participants in chat rooms or using social media that is not properly secured and protected may have a false sense that their identities are not available to other participants.

Adverse Use. Several studies have voiced concerns that participants engaged in interventions may use computers for alternative purposes. For example, online interventions using chat rooms have been used by participants to solicit sex. This is especially concerning for interventions targeted at adolescents.

Cost to Participants. Not all intervention programs can afford to provide participants with necessary intervention technologies (e.g., mobile phones, Internet). As such, participants

Concerns	Example
Literacy	• Use of websites and text messaging requires a basic level of computer literacy and reading level. • Participants may not understand health information and take adverse actions based on misunderstanding. • Participants who take online risk screening may have a false sense of safety regarding their risks.
Confidentiality	• Confidential health information cannot be transmitted on the Internet in some settings. • Other persons may gain access to a mobile device and read text messages with sensitive information. • Participants may disclose personal information on the Internet.
Adverse Use	• Participants may misuse online chat rooms or social media sites for soliciting sex, selling drugs or other illegal trade. • Adolescents may engage in inappropriate activities or be solicited.
Cost to Participants	• While mobile devices may be inexpensive, services required (e.g., Internet access, mobile cell service providers) to use such devices is still relatively costly. • Mobile devices are transitional; participants change providers and phone numbers frequently making prolonged contact challenging.
Cost of Technology and Application Development	• Providers may need to invest considerable costs in the development of web-based interventions or other content ("Apps"). • Providers may need to train staff to implement and utilize the technologies.
Replacement of the Human Factor	• The impact of substituting a computer for a person conducting an intervention is unknown; removing the human factor from the intervention may not be effective in all settings or for all participants.
Digital Divide	• While the use of computer, Internet and mobile phones is increasing for all populations, there remains a considerably large number of individuals within target populations for HIV prevention and testing who do not have access to these technologies.

Table 2. Examples of concerns related to the use of technologies to promote health.

may need to pay for monthly mobile phone or Internet access in order to remain a participant in the intervention. Well-intended participants may withdraw from an intervention solely because they cannot afford the required technology, thus continuous contact with participants may become challenging for intervention providers.

Cost of Technology and Application Development. While there are savings associated with the use or incorporation of technologies, there are also costs related to the purchase of computers, design of websites, and programming of software applications. Further, there may also be costs associated with the training needs of staff using or implementing the technologies. Some uses of technologies may require the need for additional staff. For instance, additional staff may be needed to monitor chat rooms and social media sites.

Replacement of the Human Factor. The vast majority of evidence-based interventions to reduce HIV risk and increase testing have been designed to be delivered by human interventionists. Much is yet to be learned about the efficacy of replacing humans with technology-based intervention platforms. Future research is clearly needed to examine what benefits or shortfalls emerge when an intervention is delivered solely by a computer or mobile device devoid of personal contact.

Digital Divide. Despite the growing use of and reliance on technologies by society, some populations do not have access to it. This is especially notable among the very poorest populations (National Telecommunications and Information Administration and US Department of Commerce, 1999). Interventions targeting such populations will need to be provided to participants or available to participants in convenient locations.

5. Future directions

It will be important for future research to address research questions related to the use of technologies to increase HIV testing and reduce HIV/AIDS in at-risk populations. The majority of work to date has been on MSM; little is known about how interventions should be developed differently across populations or for those who lack computer skills. Further, few studies have examined the lasting impact of technology-based interventions or the ability to maintain contact with clients over time when interventions utilize these technologies.

Our review of the literature for this chapter did not reveal any "bundled" HIV intervention approaches that examine the efficacy of combining in-person and computer-based interaction in an intervention. Measuring the efficacy of the technology-based interventions as compared to traditional in-person approaches is in early stages, and rarely have studies been conducted comparing human-administered intervention to the same content delivered by a computer or a mobile phone. There may well be target populations for whom such technology-based approaches are not appropriate.

One thing is for certain, the technologies available for use in HIV-related interventions increases daily. There are new mobile devices with new "Apps" emerging all the time and the use statistics indicate that virtually everyone will eventually have some access to computers and/or mobile devices, even in remote countries around the world. The ability to examine such interventions with different target populations in different cultural contexts opens a new world for health education and interventions. There is a need for information regarding the barriers and facilitators to adoption of technologies for HIV-specific programs.

There is also a need for more information on the capacity of organizations to implement technologies in place of more traditional approaches. In this new era of technology-based interventions for HIV prevention, the only thing that remains certain is that opportunities to apply these technologies will grow much more quickly than our ability to understand all of the implications.

6. References

Alemagno, S.A., Stephens, R.C., Stephens, P., Shaffer-King, M.A., White, P. (2009). Brief motivational intervention to reduce HIV risk and to increase HIV testing among offenders under community supervision. *Journal of Correctional Health Care, 15(3),* 210-221.

Blas, M.M., Alva, I.E., Cabello, R., Garcia, P.J., Carcamo, C., Redmon, M., Kimball, A.M., Ryan, R., & Kurth, A.E. (2007). Internet as a tool to access high-risk men who have sex with men from a resource-constrained setting: A study from Peru. *Sexually Tranmitted Infections, 83,* 567-570.

Booth, A.O., Nowson, C.A., & Matters, H. (2008). Evaluation of an interactive, Internet-based weight loss program: A pilot study. *Health Education Research, 23,* 371-381.

Bowen, A.M., Williams, M.L., Daniel, C.M., & Clayton, S. (2008). Internet based HIV prevention research targeting rural MSM: feasibility, acceptability, and preliminary efficacy. *Journal of Behavioral Medicine, 31,* 463-477.

Brendryen, H., & Kraft, P. (2008). A randomized controlled trial of a digital multi-media smoking cessation intervention. *Addiction, 103,* 478-484.

Bull, S.S., Phibbs, S., Watson, S., & McFarlane, M. (2007). What do young adults expect when they go online? Lessons for development of an STD/HIV and pregnancy prevention website. *Journal of Medical Systems, 31,* 149-158.

Bull, S. (2011). Technology-Based Health Promotion. Thousand Oaks, CA: Sage Publications.

Centers for Disease Control and Prevention. (2010, July). *HIV/AIDS.* Retrieved June 15, 2011, from http://www.cdc.gov/hiv/

Centers for Disease Control and Prevention. (2003). MMWR, *52(15).*

Centers for Disease Control and Prevention. (2001). MMWR, *50(RR19).*

Centers for Disease Control and Prevention. (2006). MMWR, Released Recommendations for HIV Testing of Adults, Adolescents, and Pregnant Women in Health Care Settings.

Chiasson, M., Hirshfield, S., & Rietmeijer, C. (2010, December 15). HIV Prevention and Care in the Digital Age. *Journal of Acquired Immune Deficiency Syndromes, 55*(2), S94-S97.

Connell, S., Sanders, M. R., & Markie-Dadds, C. (1997). Self-directed behavioral family intervention for parents of oppositional children in rural and remote areas. *Behavior Modification, 21,* 379-408.

Cullen, K.W., Thompson, D. 2008. Feasibility of an 8-week African American web-based pilot program promoting healthy eating Behaviors: Family Eats. American Journal of Health Behavior. 32(1):40-51.

DeLeon, P. H., Wakefield, M., & Hagglund, K. J. (2003). The behavioral health care needs of rural communities in the 21st century. In H. B. Stamm (Ed.), *Rural behavioral health care: An interdisciplinary guide* (pp. 23-32). Washington, DC: American Psychological Association.

Feldacker, C., Torrone, E., Triplette, M., Smith, J. C., & Leone, P. A. (2010). Reaching and Retaining High-Risk HIV/AIDs Clients Through the Internet. *Health Promotion Practice*, 522-528.

Glasgow, R.E., Klesges, L.M., Dzewaltowski, D.A., Estabrooks, P.A., & Vogt, T.M. (2006). Evaluating the impact of health promotion programs: Using the RE-AIM framework to form summary measures for decision making involving complex issues. *Health Education Research, 21,* 688-694.

Glasgow, R.E., Lichtenstein, E., & Marcus, A.C. (2003). Why don't we see more translation of health promotion research to practice? Rethinking the efficacy-to-effectiveness transition. *American Journal of Public Health, 93,* 1261-1267.

Grimley, D.M., & Hook, E.W. (2009). A 15-minute interactive, computerized condom use intervention with biological endpoints. *Sexually Transmitted Diseases, 36(2),* 73-78.

Haberer, J. E., Kwianuka, J., Nansera, D., Wilson, I. B., & Bangsberg, D. B. (2010). Challenges in Using Mobile Phones for Collection of Antiretroviral Therapy Adherence Data in a Resource-Limitied Setting. *AIDS Behavior, 14,* 1294-1301.

Hightow-Weidman, L. B., Fowler, B., Kibe, J., McCoy, R., Pike, E., Calabria, M., et al. (2011). HEALTHMPOWERMENT.ORG: Development of a Theory-Based HIV/STI Website for Young Black MSM. *AIDS Education and Prevention, 23*(1), 1-12.

Hollon, S., Munoz, R., Barlow, D., Beardslee, W., Bell, C., & Bernal, G. (2002). Psychosocial intervention development for the prevention and treatment of depression: Promoting innovation and increasing access. *Biological Psychiatry, 52,* 610-630.

Holt, M., Rawstorne, P., Wilkinson, J., Worth, H., Bittman, M., & Kippax, S. HIV Testing, Gay Community Involment and Internet USE: Social and Behavioural Correlates of HIV Tersting Among Australian Men Who Have Sex with Men. *AIDS and Behavior,* DOI: 10.1007/s10461-010-9872-z [published Online First: 7 January 2011].

Hou, S.-I., & Luh, W.-M. (2007, June). The Structure of a Web-Based HIV Testing Belief Inventory (wHITBI) for College Students: the Evidence of Construct Validation. *Medical Informatics and the Internet in Medicine,* 83-92.

Jerant, A., Sohler, N., Fiscella, K., Franks, B., & Franks, P. (2010). Tailored interactive multimedia computer programs to reduce health disparities: Opportunities and challenges. *Patient education and counseling,* 1-8. Elsevier Ireland Ltd. doi: 10.1016/j.pec.2010.11.012.

Juzang, I., Fortune, T., Black, S., Wright, E., & Bull, S. (2011, January 26). A Pilot Programme Using Mobile Phones for HIV Prevention. *Journal of Telemedicine and Telecare,* 150-153.

Kaiser Family Foundation. (2006, September). *HIV/AIDS.* Retrieved June 15, 2011, from The Kaiser Family Foundation: http://www.kff.org/hivaids/

Klesges, L., Estabrooks, P., Dzewaltowski, D., Bull, S., & Glosgow, R.E. (2007). Beginning with the application of the mind: Designing and planning health behavior change interventions to enhance dissemination. *Annals of Behavioral Medicine, 29,* 6675.

Kreuter, M., Farrell, D., Olevitch, L., & Brennan, L. (2000). Tailoring health messages: Customizing communication with computer technology. Mahwah, NJ: Erlbaum.

Lau, J., Thomas, J., & Liu, J. L. (2000, June 16). Moblie Phone and Interactive Computer Interviewing to Measure HIV-Related Risk Behaviours: the Impacts of Data Collection Methods on Research Results. *AIDS, 14*(9), 1277.

Lau, J., Tsui, H., & Wang, Q. (2003). Effects of Two Telephone Survey Methods on the Level of Reported Risk Behaviours. *Sexually Transmitted Infections, 79,* 325-331.

Leeman-Castillo, B.F., Beaty, B.F., Raghunath, S.F.A., Steiner, J., Steiner, J.F., & Bull, S. (2010). LUCHAR: Using computer technology to battle heart disease among Latinos. *American Journal of Public Health, 100,* 272-275.

Magee, J. C., Bigelow, L., DeHaan, S., & Mustanski, B. S. (2011, April 13). Sexual Health Information Seeking Online: A Mixed-Methods Study Among Lesbian, Gay, Bisexual, and Transgender Young People. *Health Education & Behavior*, 1-14.

Marks, G., et al. (2005). Meta-analysis of high-risk sexual behavior in persons aware and unaware they are infected with HIV in the United States: Implications for HIV prevention programs. *Journal of AIDS, 39(4).*

Miyazaki, M., Stuart, M., Liu, L., Tell, S., & Stewart, M. (2003). Use of ISDN video-phones for clients receiving palliative and antenatal home care. *Journal of Telemedicine and Telecare, 9,* 72-77.

National Institute of Mental Health. (2003). *Internet-based research interventions in mental health: How are they working?* Washington, DC.

National Telecommunications and Information Administration and US Department of Commerce. (1999). *Falling through the Net III: Defining the Digital Divide.*

Noar, S. (2011, May). Computer Technology-Based Intervetnions in HIV prevention: State of the Evidence and Future Directions for Research. *AIDS Care, 23*(5), 525-533.

Noar, S. M., Black, H. G., & Pierce, L. B. (2009). Efficacy of Computer Technology-Based HIV Prevention Interventions: a Meta-Analysis. *AIDS, 23,* 107-115.

Noar, S. M., Webb, E. M., Van Stee, S. K., Redding, C. A., Feist-Price, S., Crosby, R., et al. (2011, January 21). Using Computer Technology for HIV Prevntion Among African-Americans: Development of a Tailored Information Program for Safe Sex. *Health Education Research, 26*(3), 393-406.

Nordal, K. C., Copans, S. A., & Stamm, H. B. (2003). Children and adolescents in rural and frontier areas. In H. B. Stamm (Ed.), *Rural behavioral health care: An interdisciplinary guide* (pp. 159-170). Washington, DC: American Psychological Association.

Organista, K. C., Munoz, R. F., & Gonzalez, G. (1994). Cognitive-behavioral therapy for depression in low-income and minority medical outpatients: Description of a program and exploratory analyses. *Cognitive Therapy and Research, 18*(3), 241-259.

Owens, S. L., Arora, N., Quinn, N., Peeling, R. W., Holmes, K. K., & Gaydos, C. A. (2009, October 22). Utilising the Internet to Test for Sexually Transmitted Infections: Results of a Survey and Accuracy Testing. *Sexually Transmitted Infections, 86,* 112-116.

Person, A., Blain, M., Jiang, H., Rasmussen, P., & Stout, J. (2011). Text Messaging for Enhancement of Testing and Treatment for Tuberculosis, Human Immunodefiency Virus, and Syphilis: a Survey of Attitudes Toward Cellular Phones and Healthcare. *Telemedicine and e-Health, 17*(3), 189-195.

Pop-Eleches, C., Thirumurthy, H., Habyarimana, J. P., Zivin, J. G., Goldstein, M. P., Damien de Walque, et al. (2011). Moblie phone technologies improve adherence to antiretroviral treatment in a resource-limited setting: A randomized controlled trial of text message reminders. *AIDS, 25(6),* 825-34.

Rainie, L., Horrigan, J., Wellman, B., & Boase, J. (2006). *The strength of Internet ties.* Retrieved April 25, 2011 from http://www.pewinternet.org/Reports/2006/The-Strength-of-Internet-Ties.aspx.

Rhodes, S. D., Vissman, A. T., Stowers, J., Miller, C., McCoy, T. P., Hergenrather, K. C., et al. (2011). A CBPR Partnership Increases HIV Testing Among Men Who Have Sex with Men (MSM): Outcome Findings from a Pilot Test of the CyBER/testing Internet Intervention. *Health Education & Behavior, 38*(3), 311-320.

Rice, E., Monro, W., Barman-Adikari, A., & Young, S. D. (2010). Internet Use, Social Networking, and HIV/AIDS Risk for Homeless Adolescents. *Journal of Adolescent Health, 47*, 610-613.

Samal, L., Saha, S., Chander, G., Korthuis, P. T., Sharma, R. K., Sharp, V., et al. (2011). Internet Health Information Seeking Behavior and Antiretroviral Adnerence in Persons Living with HIV/AIDS. *AIDS Patient Care and STDs, 25*(7), 445-449.

Skinner, D., Rivette, U., & Bloomberg, C. (2007). Evaluation of use of cellphones to aid compliance with drug therapy for HIV patients. *AIDS Care: Psychological and Socio-medical Aspects of AIDS/HIV, 19(5)*, 605-607.

Stamm, H. B. (2003). *Rural behavioral health care: An interdisciplinary guide*. Washington, DC: American Psychological Association.

Strecher, V.J. (1999). Computer-tailored smoking cessation materials: A review and discussion. *Patient Education and Counseling, 36*, 107-117.

Stupiansky, N. W., Rosenberger, J. G., Schick, V., Herbenick, D., Novak, D. S., & Reece, M. (2010). Factors Associated with Sexually Transmitted Infection Testing Among Men who Utilize an Internet-Based Men Who Have Sex With Men Community. *AIDS Patient Care and STDs, 24(11)*, 1-5.

Sugrue, M., & Riggs, V. (2005). "Can you see and hear me now?" The implementation of camera phones in the home care setting. *Home Health Care Management & Practice, 17*, 192-195.

Swendeman, D., & Rotheram-Borus, M. (2010, March). Innovation in Sexually Transmitted Disease and HIV Prevention: Internet and Mobile Phone Delivery Vehicles for Global Diffusion. *Curr Opin Psychiatry, 23*(2), 139-144.

Thyrian, J.R., & Ulrich, J. (2007). Population impact--Definition, calculation and its use in prevention science in the example of tobacco smoking reduction. *Health Policy, 82*, 348-356.

US Census Bureau. (2002). *Health insurance coverage: 2001*. Washington, DC.

Weismann, M. M., & Jensen, P. (2002). What research suggests for depressed women with children. *Journal of Clinical Psychology, 63*(7), 614-647.

Whiteley, L. B., Brown, L. K., Swenson, R. R., Romer, D., DiClemente, R. J., Salzar, L. F., et al. (2011). African American Adolescents and New Media: Associations with HIV/STI Risk Behavior and Psychosocial Variables. *Ethnicity & Disease, 21*(Spring), 216-222.

World Health Organization. (2009). *2009 AIDS Epidemic Update.* Retrieved June 15, 2011, from UNAIDS: http://www.unaids.org/en/media/unaids/contentassets/dataimport/pub/report/2009/jc1700_epi_update_2009_en.pdf

World Health Organization. (2009). *Epidemiology.* Retrieved June 15, 2011, from UNAIDS: http://www.unaids.org/en/dataanalysis/epidemiology/

Young, S. D., & Rice, E. (2011, September 17). Online Social Networking Technologies, HIV Knowedge, and Sexual Risk and Testing Behaviors Among Homeless Youth. *AIDS Behavior, 15*, 253-260.

Zablotska, I. B., Holt, M., & Prestage, G. (2011, March 19). Changes in Gay Men's Participation in Gay Community Life: Implications for HIV Surveillance and Research. *AIDS Behavior.*

Zeanah, P., Stafford, B., & Zeanah, C. (2005). *Clinical interventions to enhance infant mental health: A selective review*. Los Angeles.

Part 2

Epidemiology and HIV Infection

4

"Bringing Testing to the People": A Discussion of an HIV-Testing Outreach Project Targeting Impoverished Women

L.R. Norman[1], B. Williams[2], R. Rosenberg[3], C. Alvarez-Garriga[1], L. Cintron[1] and R. Malow[3]

[1]Ponce School of Medicine and Health Sciences, Ponce,
[2]Jackson State University, Jackson, Mississippi,
[3]Florida International University, Miami, FL,
[1]Puerto Rico
[2,3]United States

1. Introduction

1.1 Health disparities related to HIV

HIV-related health disparities are differences in the incidence, prevalence, mortality, and/or burden of HIV and related adverse health conditions that exist among specific population groups. Health disparities exist within the impoverished or low-income housed population in Puerto Rico with respect to HIV. Formative research findings with women who live in public housing revealed a three percent self-reported HIV positive serostatus (Norman, et. al., 2008). However, due to the stigma associated with HIV in Puerto Rico, especially within the residents of public housing, this figure is likely to be an underestimation of the real seroprevalence (Norman, et. al., 2009). The vast majority is unemployed (95%) and has no visible means of monetary support. As such, they qualify for "Reform, as the local Puerto Rico Health Reform program (*Reforma de Salud de Puerto Rico* in Spanish), is called. This is a government-run program which provides medical and healthcare services to indigent and impoverished citizens of Puerto Rico. It is run by means of contracting services of private health insurance companies, as opposed to the traditional system of government-owned hospitals and emergency centers. The Reform is administered by the Puerto Rico Health Insurance Administration and, as of December 31, 2005, provides healthcare coverage to over 1.5 million Puerto Ricans, which equals to 37.5% of the island population (PR Department of Health, 2010). While these persons qualify for Reform, many of them have no means of accessing needed health care due to the costs of or lack of transportation.

The course of HIV disease varies among individuals, with complications such as opportunistic infections (OIs) emerging at different times throughout the trajectory of the illness. The goal of healthcare is to keep the individual as healthy as possible through health-promoting behaviors. When examining the quality of life among PR residents, one study found that older women, persons with less education or *lower income*, persons unable to work, and those who were overweight or who had diabetes or high blood pressure reported more days for which they were physically or mentally unhealthy during the 30 days preceding the survey (CDC, 2002). Health-promoting behaviors include good nutrition and ongoing risk reduction, as well as making persons aware of their HIV status. Ensuring that people know their HIV status and receive adequate care if infected can improve clinical outcomes and reduce the transmission of HIV. However, researchers estimate that 21 percent of persons infected with HIV are unaware that they have the disease (IOM 2011). Once persons are made aware of their positive status, they can be offered treatment and appropriate care, which can help decrease HIV-related disparities associated with morbidity and mortality.

1.2 Why impoverished females in Puerto Rico are considered disproportionately affected by HIV/AIDS

As of September 2011, 43,648 cases of AIDS have been reported in the island (PR Department of Health, 2011). Women constitute 20% of the total number of prevalent cases. Heterosexual transmission accounts for 61% of the cases among women, followed by injecting drug use (IDU) (PR Department of Health, 2011).

Puerto Rico has one of the highest incidence rates of AIDS in the Americas (CDC, 2010). In the year 2009, rates of HIV diagnoses among female adults and adolescents ages 13 years and older in Puerto Rico had then 5th highest rates among 40 states and five US territories, with a rate of 15.4 cases per 100,000 population (CDC, 2010). Prevalence rates of adult and adolescent females living with a diagnosis of HIV infection, year-end 2008, revealed that Puerto Rico was the 3rdn highest, with 349.7 cases per 100,000 population. Lastly, in terms of rates of AIDS diagnosis among adult and adolescent females in 2009, Puerto Rico reported the 5th highest rate with 13.2 cases per 100,000 population being reported.

The estimated HIV prevalence was calculated for women and girls living in Puerto Rico using the data described above and the population of Puerto Rico residents, which includes approximately 3.8 million, of which approximately 1.6 million are female aged 13 years and older (US Census Bureau, 2011). At the end of 2008, the estimated prevalence among women and girls ages 13 years and older living in Puerto Rico was 69 cases per 10,000 women (0.69 per 100) (CDC, 2010). While this prevalence rate may seem to be low, self-reported data collected from 1,138 women during the formative phase of *Proyecto MUCHAS* revealed a rate more than four times that estimate, with three percent self-reporting their HIV status as positive (Norman, et. al., 2008). This rate does not include those women who refused to disclose their status on the survey. If we include assume they are positive and include them, the rate goes up to 3.9 per 100. As the percentage of AIDS cases among women continues to increase in Puerto Rico, it becomes imperative that research and prevention efforts target additional groups of women who may be at increased risk of HIV.

1.3 Social and cultural factors that exacerbate HIV risk for impoverished women

HIV risks are exacerbated for impoverished women by a number of social and cultural factors. Poverty is a major factor that contributes to the increased risk of HIV for women. Many experts believe poverty, unemployment, and a lack of education are helping to drive the growing HIV problem among women. Women living in inner-city poor neighborhoods are often in poor health and without access to healthcare for prevention or treatment (Women's Health, 2011). While risky behaviors in these communities directly spread HIV, urban poverty is clearly playing an important role because it is directly related to lack of or low education, poor housing conditions, and other factors associated to low self-esteem, and lack of knowledge about health issues. Previous research has examined the relationship between socioeconomic status and HIV risk and identifying significant associations between the two, such as persons who are considered low-income are more likely to be HIV positive than are their higher income peers (CDC, 2011; Johns, Bauermeister, & Zimmerman, 2010; Dinkelman, Lam & Leibbrandt, 2007). The findings from these studies suggest that impoverished persons are at increased risk for HIV infection because of the heightened risk that stems from the increased HIV prevalence within their social/sexual networks. Furthermore, the physical, psychological, and social circumstances in which their poverty places them may also increase their risk of HIV exposure.

In addition to the risk that poverty imposes on impoverished women, another social issue contributing to increased risk for women and girls has to do with gender socialization (Carovano, 1992). *Gender* refers to the widely shared expectations and norms held by a society with regard to appropriate male and female behavior, characteristics, and roles. It is a social and cultural construct that differentiates women from men and defines the ways in which women and men interact with each other (Carovano, 1992). With respect to women's vulnerability, in many societies, there is a culture of silence surrounding sex that dictates that "good" women are expected to be ignorant about sex and passive in sexual interactions, making it difficult for women to be well informed about risk reduction or, even when informed, making it difficult for them to be proactive in negotiating safer sex with their male partners (Carovano, 1992). The women in the above mentioned study sample of Puerto Rican residents are members of just such a society. Another issue related to this culture in many societies is the belief that variety in sexual partners is essential to men's nature as men, and that men need to seek multiple partners for sexual release; the manifestations of traditional notions of masculinity are strongly associated with a wide range of risk-taking behaviors among men that affect both men and women (Courtney, 1998).

Research with impoverished minority women suggests that these women who live in male-dominated societies are at a significant risk of HIV due to increased levels of drug use, risky sexual practices, and intimate partner violence, among other factors; in addition, there may be significant levels of interaction with members of concentrated groups (Fuller, et. al., 2005; Brown-Peterside, et. al., 2002; Kalichman, et. al., 1998; Soler, et. al., 2000) While current research findings can be used to hypothesize increased HIV risk, data on impoverished Latina women in Puerto Rico are scarce, so it is difficult to estimate either the levels of HIV risk or the factors contributing to such risk for this population. Unique cultural and social factors may exist, which contribute significantly to the exacerbation of HIV and STIs risk for impoverished Latina women living in public housing developments of Puerto Rico.

As is frequently the case in Latino societies, children born into the Puerto Rican culture find themselves subjected to attitudes, mores, and customs that promote very strong gender differences. From birth on, these differences are inherent in every aspect of sexual expression and male-female interaction (Raffaelli, 2004). The outward manifestation of the principle illustrated by these differences is called *machismo*, which is the belief that males are physically, intellectually, culturally, and sexually superior to females. Because of this pervasive attitude, women are relegated to the role of being sexual objects with the sole aim of fulfilling men's desires and needs (Montesinos & Preciado, 2001). Furthermore, in Puerto Rico, these ideas are prevalent among members of the low-income population, who tend to agree with the more traditional values as related to gender (Pico, 1998). These factors need to be considered if one is to develop culturally appropriate, effective interventions to decrease HIV/STI risk-related behaviors among these women.

Therefore, research into HIV-prevention efforts needs to explore the mechanisms by which various social and cultural constructs increase women's vulnerability to HIV. By developing an understanding of these constructions, one can begin to develop and implement appropriate and effective strategies to improve women's situations. Given the patterns and inequalities in the roles of women and men, it is not surprising that women are at high risk for HIV transmission, especially those who live in societies that are impoverished and that support male dominance over women as well as gender inequality. Furthermore, considering these additional cultural and social factors present in Puerto Rico, impoverished women who live in a male dominated society may be at a significantly higher risk for HIV than are their peers who do not live in such a society.

1.4 Importance of HIV testing

Public HIV antibody testing started in 1985 and two years later, was expanded. This expansion included the development of voluntary counseling and testing (VCT) guidelines, due to the new treatment discovery (i.e., Retrovir [AZT, Zidovudine]), which was approved by the FDA and offered to those individuals who tested positive for HIV (Cichocki, 2010). As such, since treatment has become available, it is standard procedure to offer VCT to any person seeking HIV testing. This allows for persons testing positive for HIV to learn how to modify their behavior to reduce the risk of HIV transmission to others; as well as providing the linkage medical care and services that further reduce morbidity, mortality, and improve quality of life. Today, HIV testing is almost standard operating procedure in all of the following: urgent care clinics, inpatient services, substance abuse treatment clinics, public health clinics, community clinics, correctional health-care facilities, and primary care settings. Conventional tests such as the ELISA antibody test take up to a week to complete, which lessens the likelihood that patients return for the results. In addition to the lengthy process for awaiting results, other barriers include fear of the testing results, denial that they have been exposed to HIV, an assumption that they are HIV-negative, the ramifications of an HIV-positive result, ignorance about treatment, fear of discrimination, and perceived stigma (Galvin et al., 2000).

1.5 Introduction to rapid HIV testing

Initially, conventional tests such as the ELISA and Western Blot tests were the gold standard of HIV testing. Conventional tests still play a vital role in HIV testing but current rapid HIV testing provides a less intrusive modality for determining a person's HIV status. However, it is recommended that a positive rapid HIV test result be followed up with confirmatory testing, such as the ELISA and Western Blot as described above because it is believed that confirmatory blood testing with more sophisticated testing algorithms are more accurate. Recommendations for HIV testing in health care settings, published by the Centers for Disease Control and Prevention (CDC), have led to increased rapid HIV testing in a variety of settings including emergency departments (Haukoos et al., 2011). In 2003, CDC introduced an initiative to reduce barriers to early diagnosis of HIV infection and increase access to treatment and prevention services entitled, "Advancing HIV Prevention: New Strategies for a Changing Epidemic" (AHP). The initiative placed an emphasis on offering routine HIV testing as part of the medical visit. It also highlighted the importance of using rapid HIV tests to facilitate access to early diagnosis in high prevalence areas (CDC, 2003; Greenwald et al., 2006). The initiative promotes four strategies: (1) make HIV testing a routine part of medical care; (2) prevent new infections by working with persons diagnosed with HIV and their partners; (3) further decrease mother-to-child HIV transmission; and, (4) implement new models for diagnosing HIV infections outside medical settings. In particular, the latter strategy funded new demonstration projects using OraQuick® to increase access to early diagnosis and referral for treatment and prevention services in high-HIV prevalence settings. It created new prospects for expanding HIV testing to identify and treat HIV-infected persons earlier in the progression of the disease than ever before.

Rapid HIV tests can provide results in as little as 10 minutes, depending on the test. Persons receiving reactive test results from the initial testing visit are left with information indicative that they are highly likely to be seropositive compared with receiving no test information at the end of the visit where a conventional HIV test specimen was collected (Greenwald et al., 2006). The five FDA-approved rapid HIV tests include OraQuick Advance Rapid HIV-1/2 Antibody Test (finger prick; venipuncture whole blood, serum, plasma; oral fluid); Reveal Rapid HIV-1 Antibody Test (serum, plasma); Uni-Gold Recombigen HIV Test (serum, plasma, venipuncture whole blood); Multispot HIV-1/HIV-2 Rapid Test (serum, plasma) (Kaiser Foundation, 2005) and Clearview 1/2 Stat-Pak and Clearview Complete HIV ½ (Whole blood, serum/plasma) (Pacific AIDS Education and Training Center, 2009).

Similar to conventional HIV tests, reactive rapid HIV tests require confirmation. Among all rapid HIV tests, the commonalities include the process in which the tests functions (i.e., visual interpretation, lack of instrumentation, and affixation of HIV antigens to the test strip or membrane), the periodic use of external controls (i.e., known HIV-positive and -negative specimens), the use of product information sheets that are provided to the patients, and confirmation by a more specific assay (Western Blot or immunofluorescent assay) for reactive results (Greenwald et al., 2006).

1.6 Participant satisfaction with rapid HIV testing

There are tremendous advantages to using rapid HIV testing, as discussed earlier, compared to conventional HIV tests. Patient satisfaction has played an integral role to sustaining the implementation of CDC's recommended HIV screening for patients in all health care settings. It enhances that: (1) patients with newly identified infection learn the importance of seeking immediate care; and (2) patients at high risk of infection continue to be open to appropriate retesting (Donnell-Fink et al., 2011). Thus, a number of studies have been conducted to determine patient satisfaction with rapid HIV testing in a variety of settings and programs.

One of the earliest studies was conducted by Spielberg et al. (2003). A survey of elicited testing motivators, barriers, and preferences for new strategies was administered to a sample of 460 participants at the following: a needle exchange, three sex venues for men who have sex with men, and a sexually transmitted disease clinic. It was found that most of the participants preferred rapid testing strategies (clinic-based and home self-testing).

Two years later, Spielberg et al. (2005) did further research to show that rapid HIV testing is overwhelmingly preferred by people seeking to know their status. In a randomized study involving the selection of alternative HIV counseling and testing approaches based on the results of focus groups and interviews, a preference survey administered to clients at the three study sites in Seattle (i.e., a needle exchange program and two bathhouses frequented by MSM), found that in outreach settings, alternative HIV counseling and testing strategies help to maximize the number of clients who learn their HIV test results. Furthermore, it was found that traditional HIV testing with standard counseling was least effective at providing clients with knowledge of their HIV status. Significantly more participants chose to learn their HIV serostatus based on a variety of advantages that included offering a combination of rapid oral fluid testing with written pretest materials. This proved the best way to increase the number of persons who learn their HIV status.

Antonio-Gaddy (2006) initiated a study at 61 HIV testing sites in New York State, comparing HIV test use during the first 6 months of rapid testing in 2003 with the same time period in 2002. Surveys were administered to clients at each site during the first 30 days of rapid testing and to counselors before and after training--and after 12 weeks of using rapid tests in the field. It was found that participants preferred finger-stick blood rapid tests (96.5%) over conventional HIV testing by drawing blood intravenously primarily because of the ability to get same-day results and a dislike of needles. Additionally, counselors reported increased self-efficacy or the perceived ability to administer the rapid test, and a heightened level of comfortableness in administering rapid HIV testing.

Donnell-Fink et al. (2011) surveyed 1,616 participants in the Universal Screening for HIV Infection in the Emergency Room (USHER) randomized controlled trial on patient satisfaction. The survey questions focused on overall satisfaction with emergency department (ED) visit, time spent on primary medical problem, time spent on HIV testing, and test provider's ability to answer HIV-related questions using a four-point Likert scale, ranging from very dissatisfied to very satisfied (defined as optimal satisfaction). It was found that, overall, 1,478 (91.5%) were very satisfied. These were the factors associated with less optimal satisfaction: reactive test result, aged 60 years or older, black race, Hispanic/Latino ethnicity, and testing by ED provider instead of HIV counselor.

Collectively, the abovementioned studies show that rapid HIV testing is in sync with CDC's recommendation for routine HIV screening and contributes to an increase in routine testing in health care settings around the world. The factors associated with patient satisfaction are important.

1.7 Challenges of rapid HIV testing

Essentially, rapid HIV tests are screening tests that require confirmation by Western Blot or Immunofluorescence antibody, which are more specific assays. Consequently, a reactive or positive test result is considered a preliminary positive. Though highly unlikely (2%), false-positives do occur with rapid HIV testing, at slightly higher rates than the confirmatory testing, mainly as a result of medical conditions such as Hepatitis A and B viruses (Greenwald et al., 2006).

Over the past few years, several studies have been done to examine sensitivity and specificity issues associated with rapid HIV tests. Tests that require the use of oral fluid, such as OraQuick, have been found to be most at risk of false positives. Delaney et al., (2006) compared the accuracy of the rapid test performed on whole blood and oral fluid specimens with the results of conventional HIV tests by using four separate studies, in which all participants were provided oral fluid, fingerstick or anticoagulated whole blood specimens for testing with OraQuick (on both oral fluid and whole blood). Though it was found that the OraQuick test demonstrated high sensitivity and specificity for HIV antibody with both whole blood and oral fluid specimens, OraQuick sensitivity (99.1% vs. 99.6%) and specificity (99.6% vs. 99.7%) were lower with oral fluid than with whole blood. This small amount of difference becomes important with dealing with large populations tested.

A study published in *Morbidity and Mortality Weekly Report* (CDC, 2008) was published that focused on an increase in false-positives in New York clinics using oral fluid rapid tests. There were two periods of significant increases in false-positive test results over a four year span. Several months after the first increase in false-positive test results during late 2005, oral fluid testing in clinics was suspended (3 weeks) and replaced with finger-stick whole-blood rapid testing, which produced no false-positive test results. After the second increase in November 2007, the New York City Department of Health and Mental Hygiene halted all oral fluid testing in favor of finger-stick whole blood specimens. However ultimately, the performance of oral fluid rapid tests still exceeded the Food and Drug Administration's minimum threshold of 98.0% specificity and, the authors that use of oral rapid tests makes HIV testing possible in many venues where performing phlebotomy or finger sticks is impractical for screening.

1.8 Impact of cultural differences on HIV rapid testing

It is reasonable to assume that the knowledge, beliefs, and attitudes about HIV testing are similar among all cultures. Persons living with HIV are stigmatized, ostracized, stereotyped, and shunned, regardless of the culture. The attitudes toward HIV testing appear to be slightly different. The failure to use HIV testing services by significant numbers of individuals at risk for HIV can be attributed to a number of factors, both on an individual as well as a societal level. Research has shown that the reasons high-risk Americans avoid HIV testing include fear of learning they are HIV-positive, belief that they are unlikely to have been exposed to HIV, belief that they are HIV-negative, the possibility of being HIV-positive, the assumption that there is little they can do about being HIV-positive, perceived stigma, and fear (Galvin, 2000; Samet, 1997).

It appears that the aforementioned reasons are not necessarily the same for other countries. Peltzer et al. (2004) sought to determine the attitudes of HIV testing and determinants of attitudes toward persons living with HIV (PLWH) among 600 first-year university students from South India, South Africa and America--vis-à-vis a self-administered questionnaire. It was found that American students had much more positive attitudes toward HIV testing than South African and Indian students. Statistical analyses showed that attitudes toward HIV testing were correlated, for instance, with contact readiness, which refers to the degree to which a person is ready to be within close proximity of a person living with HIV (PLWHs). Positive HIV testing attitudes were positively correlated with contact readiness with PLWHs, for instance.

In the Caribbean, culture has played and continues to play a large role in HIV testing acceptance, including rapid HIV testing (Coggins, 2007). One particular aspect is that of conspiracy beliefs among African Americans and Caribbean residents alike. Many members of these populations believe that HIV/AIDS is a form of genocide against Blacks, while others feel that a cure for AIDS exists, but is being withheld from the poor. Also, a significant proportion subscribes to the beliefs that HIV/AIDS treatment professionals use people (especially minority and poor persons) as guinea pigs for the government and lastly, that AIDS is a man-made virus developed specifically targeting minority persons. These views are especially prominent within the Black community.

In sum, there are notable individual and social cultural differences in the implementation and acceptability of HIV rapid testing. Across all cultures, it is undeniable that HIV rapid testing has expanded testing opportunities in both developed and underdeveloped countries. Even as some countries continue to struggle with meager resources, feeble laboratory infrastructure, a dearth of skilled phlebotomists and technicians, and weak courier networks, HIV rapid testing is becoming more routine for high risk individuals (Scott et al., 2009).

1.9 New approaches in HIV rapid testing

Over the past decade, three landmark events have impacted the landscape of HIV rapid testing: the licensing of the first HIV rapid test approved for use with finger-stick whole blood specimens (which occurred in March 2004), the CDC's HIV prevention initiative to increase opportunities for HIV testing; and, publication of the CDC recommendations for routine screening for HIV in medical care settings. During the past few years, advances in HIV testing have resulted in the development of new strategies to increase the number of persons getting tested for HIV. These advances include the integration of HIV rapid testing in emergency departments, implementation of computer-assisted HIV rapid testing, and the use of electronic media to introduce HIV rapid testing to adolescents (CDC, 2007; Merchant et al., 2011; Calderon et al., 2011). Emergency departments (EDs) have been one of the leading venues for implementing innovative strategies to increase the uptake, feasibility and cost per outcome in HIV testing (Prabhu et al., 2011; Hutchinson et al., 2011). Despite the CDC's efforts to promote opt-out HIV screening in all EDs, it remains unavailable in several states. Psychosocial, behavioral and structural supports must be added to the HIV testing process to improve the chances of getting people tested. Merchant et al. (2011) made an unsuccessful attempt to use an audio computer-delivered tailored feedback intervention to determine if there were increases in ED patient uptake of opt-in, non-targeted rapid HIV screening. Though the intervention was not found to increase uptake in HIV testing, it showed that the belief of not being at risk for HIV (37.1%) was the most common reason for declining HIV screening, and the most common reason for accepting HIV screening was the convenience of being tested in the ED (36.8%). Moreover, it was determined that uptake is greater among patients who report more HIV risk and among those whose self-perceived HIV risk increases from baseline after completion of an HIV risk assessment.

With Apple surging past Exxon in August 2011 as the world's most valuable company, it has become clear that the most rewarding innovation is now social innovation and production that takes place on the internet. Most of what has been explored to date in HIV prevention research is limited to the use of mobile technologies as mediums for information dissemination, social marketing, or medication adherence. While there is some emerging evidence of efficacy for mobile-based HIV interventions (Swendeman & Rotheram-Borus, 2010), the new media of Web 2.0 is just beginning to be explored by HIV behavioral researchers (Bull et al., 2011; Gilliam et al., 2011). New media is defined on the AIDS.gov gateway as internet-based communication that is interactive, involving content that may be co-created and information that may be collaboratively produced on an array of digital devices. New media tools include blogs, social network sites like Facebook and Twitter, mashups, video sharing sites like Youtube, virtual worlds like Second Life, webcasts and webinars, RSS feeds and social bookmarking, wikis, podcasts, texting and mobile communication, and photo sharing sites like Flickr (see http://aids.gov/using-new-media/tools/). There are indications that social networking media could be an effective modality to removing barriers to HIV testing and reducing stigma. Calderon et al. (2011) compared the effectiveness of a youth-friendly HIV video with in-person counseling in conveying HIV knowledge and obtaining consent for HIV testing among adolescent patients of an urban ED using a convenience sample of 200 stable, sexually active people aged 15 to 21 years in an urban EDs. The results indicate that a youth-friendly HIV educational video improved adolescents' HIV knowledge and increased their participation in HIV testing more than in-person counseling. This finding is consistent with other research, including a recent meta-analysis showing that effect sizes on HIV risk indicators are similar to human-delivered interventions among 12 randomized controlled trials of internet or computer-based HIV risk reduction interventions (Noar, et. al., 2009; Swendeman & Rotheram-Borus, 2010).

An ongoing study funded by the National Institute of Nursing Research may be the first of its kind to investigate the efficacy of social media as a delivery portal for HIV prevention (Bull et al., 2011; Gilliam et al., 2011). Entitled the *Just/Us* study, the project involves a randomized trial of a Facebook intervention for youth of color. The visualization of HIV-related metrics using the internet has the potential to engage individuals outside the boundaries of traditional health care delivery and social services. The MIT Media Lab recently instituted a new research group, New Media Medicine, to discover and implement new approaches in this area. One innovation involves internet-delivered visualization of antiretroviral drug activity at the cellular level based on an individual's lab monitoring (Moss, 2011). This technology is designed to be an HIV medication adherence tool, shared between the patient and his provider.

Initiatives to increase uptake of HIV testing across various settings are continuing to be implemented by local, state, and the federal government. In 2007, the CDC expanded funding to 25 health departments in the *Expanded HIV Testing Initiative,* to enhance the obtainability and accessibility of HIV testing services, facilitate adoption of HIV screening in health-care settings, and increase identification of undiagnosed HIV infection in populations disproportionately affected by HIV (Vaill, et. al., 2011). This initiative has been enhanced to reflect key aspects of the new White House National HIV/AIDS HIV Prevention Strategy. Pivotal to the national strategy is to view HIV testing as the first step in what is frequently described as a treatment or engagement cascade. This cascade is a series of activities that are developed to make persons aware of their HIV status to linking them with care as well as adhering to their medication regime. They must be followed in sequential order to be effective (Gardner, et. al., 2011).

1.10 The role of rapid HIV testing in addressing HIV-related health disparities

The Department of Health and Human Services' Healthy People 2020 defines a health disparity as a particular type of health difference that is closely linked with social or economic disadvantage. Health disparities adversely affect groups of people who have experienced greater social or economic obstacles to health based on their racial or ethnic group, religion, socioeconomic status, ender, mental health, cognitive, sensory, or physical disability, sexual orientation, geography, or other characteristics historically linked to discrimination or exclusion. as the differences that occur by gender, race or ethnicity, education or income, disability, geographic location, or sexual orientation (U.S. Department of Health and Human Services, 2011).

In 2002, Smedley, Smith, and Nelson published a report entitled, "Unequal Treatment: Confronting Racial and Ethnic Disparities in Healthcare". The purpose of the report was to examine how bias, prejudice, and stereotyping contribute to unequal health care treatment. Among numerous findings, it was determined that there two sets of factors that contributed to disparities in health care. The first set of factors includes the operation of the healthcare systems and the legal and regulatory climate, in which they operate are significant. The second set of factors is the result of a confluence of three mechanisms: (1) bias (or prejudice) against minorities; (2) greater clinical uncertainty when interacting with minority patients; and (3) beliefs (or stereotypes) held by the provider about the behavior or health of minorities.

Minority populations typically experience higher rates of morbidity and mortality for conditions such as diabetes, cardiovascular disease, some forms of cancer and HIV/AIDS (CDC, 2005). In communities of lower socioeconomic status, the residents (i.e., gay men, drug users, prisoners and formerly incarcerated persons, the homeless, and those who suffer from a variety of mental health disabilities) are further marginalized by higher rates of HIV-related morbidity and mortality (NMAC, 2006).

CDC and other federal agencies have made tremendous strides to address health disparities in the incidence of HIV/AIDS. This has been done by prioritizing several issues: 1) enhancing and improving partnerships; 2) increasing screening and testing for diseases in populations with known health disparities; 3) adopting an integrated service model to improve health care delivery; 4) improving monitoring through the enhancement of current data systems and the development of new systems; and, 5) adopting new diagnostic, treatment, and prevention technologies (Steele et al., 2007).

CDC's 2003 "Advancing HIV Prevention" initiative focused on HIV prevention by emphasizing increased HIV testing. A number of years later, the revised recommendations for HIV testing incorporated routine opt-out HIV screening guidelines for all patients ages 13–64 in medical settings, regardless of their HIV risk. This was a considerable effort to reduce barriers to testing by eliminating previous requirements to accompany each HIV test with pretest counseling and separate written informed consent (CDC, 2006).

This initiative expanded rapid HIV testing efforts considerably. There are barriers (i.e., conflicting guidelines among federal agencies, problems with insurance coverage of routine testing, low reimbursement rates for HIV testing, and lack of programs that support clinician education and training in HIV testing) that impact the expansion of HIV testing.

However, as technology advances, new strategies are being developed that will promote expanded HIV testing, Expanding programs to notify partners of HIV-positive individuals, linking HIV testing with other health care and social services, and mounting media and social network outreach efforts are all facilitators to HIV testing, as outlined by Institute of Medicine (2011). Particularly, rapid HIV tests continue to be the preferred modality of testing by participants because the results are immediate and help reduce the number of people who fail to receive their test results. Rapid testing affords the opportunity of underserved individuals, including racial/ethnic minorities) to receive HIV testing at their home or outside of a clinic setting. Increasing the HIV testing among members of this disproportionately affected population addresses one of the top 20 priorities as outlined in *Healthy People 2020* (U.S. Department of Health and Human Services, 2011). Identifying persons who are HIV-infected and unaware of their status can lead to increasing access to care and improving health outcomes for people living with HIV, which includes a decrease in HIV-related morbidity and mortality and a better quality of life in general. This, in turns, decreases HIV-related health disparities that currently exist among members of this population.

2. A discussion of *Proyecto MUCHAS*, an HIV-testing outreach project

2.1 The inception of *Proyecto MUCHAS*

This part of the chapter will describe the development of the HIV testing outreach project targeting impoverished female residents living in public housing developments (PuHD) in Ponce, Puerto Rico (PR) entitled *Proyecto MUCHAS.* The idea for working with women unfolded in 2005, when the principal investigator (LR Norman) relocated to Ponce, PR and assumed her post at the Ponce School of Medicine and Health Sciences. In reviewing the literature of HIV preventions that had been implemented with certain sub-populations in PR, it was determined that heterosexual women, especially those impoverished, had been basically ignored. Only one study that targeted this population was found and it was conducted close to 20 years ago (Hunt, et. al., 1993). Therefore, based on previous knowledge of the increased risks that exist among members of this population documented in published research with U.S. samples, it was decided to target this population for research.

Seed money came from the Puerto Rico Comprehensive Center for HIV Disparities (PR-CCHD, NCRR Grant # U54RR19507) to conduct a two-year formative research project, which did not include HIV testing. It was started by going to the PuHD administration and getting permission and their support for research. The research team then met with the individual administrative staff at each of the PuHD we targeted during this phase (n=23 out of 25 that are managed by Machuca and Associates).

The team also decided it was important to come up with a name and a logo for the project, which would be recognizable to residents of PuHDs. The project's name became *Proyecto MUCHAS,* which stands for Proyecto - Mujeres United Combatiendo - Alerta Social. This translates into the English phrase: "Women Fighting HIV: Social Alert." Along with it, a logo was devised so that when residents see this acronym and the logo, they know it is associated with this research project (see Figure 1 below).

In addition, the research team also developed a web-page on the school's website with the above logo and a message about the goals of the project. The web address is

Fig. 1. Proyecto MUCHAS Logo

http://www.psm.edu/MUCHAS/index.htm. Lastly, the project colors are pink (both light and dark) and the logo embossed onto t-shirts, which are worn by the research team housing on the days that HIV/STI testing is being conducted.

Eligibility criteria included being female and a resident of the PuHD. A non-probability sampling approach was employed for the study (which is explained in detail below). Once a PuHD was selected, posters were placed up to announce that the project would be coming to the PuHD on a certain date and that all women were invited to come to the community center and participate in the study (See Figure 2 for Illustration of Flyer).

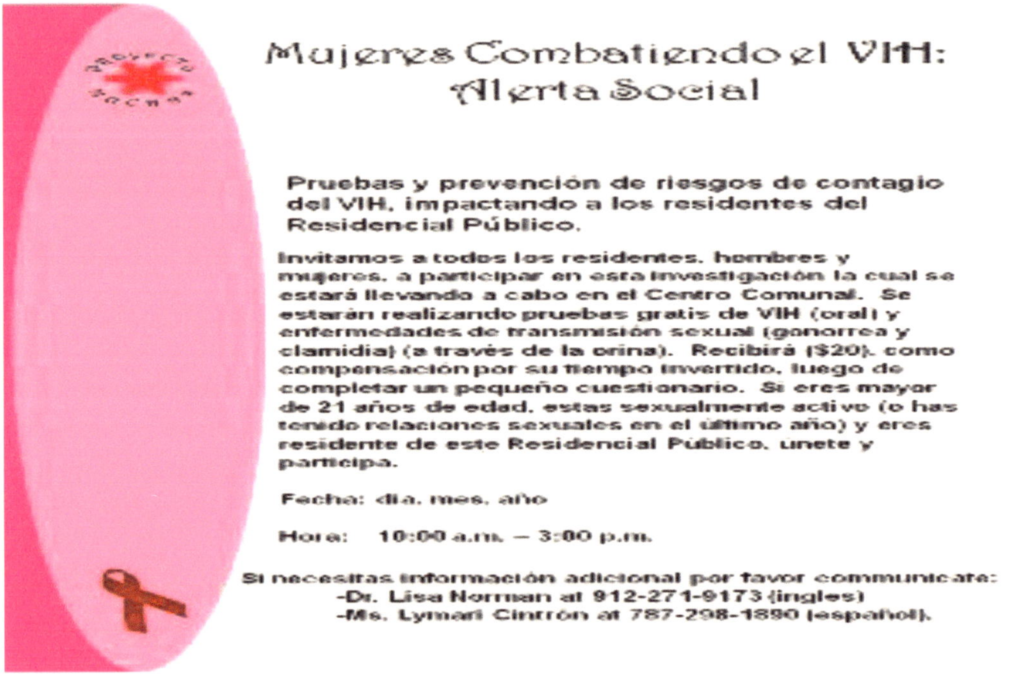

Fig. 2. Flyer Posted at PuHD to Invite Residents to Participate in *Proyecto MUCHAS.*

All eligible women were invited to participate. Data were gathered between April and August 2006 from 1138 women in 23 various PuHDs across the city of Ponce.

The research team then conducted four focus groups with 39 various members of the population at two of the large public housing developments (PuHD) (Lopez Nussa and Dr. Pila) to gather the formative data on their knowledge, perceived risks, attitudes, and behaviors related to HIV prevention. These focus groups revealed some very important information and the results were used to inform the development of a quantitative instrument. The results of the focus group have been published (Abreu, et. al., 2010). The instrument was piloted with a sample of 30 women in order to assess the ease of completing the assessment tool, to determine if the questions were easily understood, and to ensure that the instrument could be completed in a timely fashion. On the basis of the first piloting phase, revisions were made. In addition, focus groups were used to validate the instrument, with 10 female residents participating to review the quantitative assessment tool for appropriate language and content. Following the final revision, one focus group was conducted as a method to validate the survey instrument. It went over every question to make sure they were understandable and culturally appropriate. After this focus group was conducted some changes were made to the questionnaire and the version was finalized and duplicated and administered to the female residents of PuHDs. After the research team went through this time-consuming but very necessary protocol, the survey instrument was implemented to 1138 residents in the 23 PuHDs, between April and August 2006.

Women completed the assessments in the community center room within each housing development. Informed consent was received from every respondent. Because of the nature of the questions and the possible perceived threat of addressing issues related to sexual and drug-using behaviors, the instrument was self-administered with no identifiers, providing anonymity to the respondents. Research assistants provided support for those women who were unable to read the questionnaire or who needed other assistance by reading the survey to them or completing the survey on their behalf. Each woman received $10 as compensation for completing the survey. All surveys were administered in Spanish. This survey was a baseline, formative survey, occurring before any intervention or HIV-related activities were provided for the residents.

2.2 Development of *Proyecto MUCHAS* testing project

2.2.1 Prevalence of HIV among women living in Puerto Rico

Using these results and the population of Puerto Rico, as presented above, along with the self-reported HIV prevalence among female residents living in PuHDs, the research team concluded that this population was disproportionately affected by HIV. As the percentage of AIDS cases among women continues to increase in Puerto Rico, it becomes imperative that research and prevention efforts target additional groups of women who may be at increased risk of HIV.

2.2.2 Rationale for developing and implementing HIV testing out-research project

It was self-reported data that drew the research team's attention to the immediate necessity of implementing HIV testing to women who live in PuHDs (Norman, et. al., 2008). Again, as mentioned above, this self-reported rate is four times the rate of the estimated HIV prevalence among all adolescent and adult women living in Puerto Rico, according to the data provided by the Centers for Disease Control (CDC, 2010). As such, Pfizer Pharmaceuticals was approached with the data findings and they supported the project, awarding a two year contract to test 375 female residents of PuHDs.

Fortunately, by this time, the women knew who the research team was and no problems recruiting participants emerged. The team only had to visit four randomly selected PuHDs to recruit 386 women. Due to the logistics of the testing and the inability to go to the women's apartments due to safety issues, the testing had to be conducted in the community center. However, this did not deter the women from coming and participating. The research team was only able test 50 women per day, so it went to each of the four randomly selected PuHDs two times. At the present time, only two HIV positive women (2/386 = 0.01%) have been identified. The research team believes that the women who were already positive are choosing not to come because they don't see the benefit of being retested, even though STI testing (for chlamydia and gonorrhea) is offered. Consequently, the project plans to distribute additional information about the importance of retesting and STI testing in the flyers to encourage this continued participation; plans are also in place to develop information for male residents. This has not been done yet, but the plan is to go testing in the very near future to one of the largest PuHDs here in Ponce; it is one that was not visited during the formative research phase of the project.

As mentioned above, men will also be invited to participate, since 11 women tested positive for chlamydia and one tested positive for gonorrhea (2.9% and 0.03%, respectively) (Norman, et. al., 2011). It is believed that the men are the vectors of the infection for these women and, as such, the research team needs to get them tested and referred into treatment as a way to prevent further transmission to the female residents of PuHD here in Puerto Rico.

At this time, the team has not tested anyone using this new protocol. However, it is believed that the project will be successful in the continued recruitment of women as well as men in our project, if the previous success record is any indication. The project is currently funded by the RCMI program at NIH (grant # G12RR003050 awarded to the Ponce School of Medicine and Health Sciences from 2009-2014) to test another 375 residents of public housing as well as to examine the social epidemiological factors associated with the increased HIV/STI risk and prevalence among members of this population.

2.2.3 Recruitment strategies used in *Proyecto MUCHAS*

Initially, the recruitment strategies were not very effective. At the PuHD first visited (Lopez Nussa) to collect the quantitative formative data, only 15 women showed up. The research team had placed flyers up at the PuHD to announce the date coming. By this time, the logo and name were developed, as described above. Needless to say the team was very disappointed. However, a research assistant suggested the idea to use the PuHD's megaphone to drive around the complex and let the women know the team was there, and to invite them to come down and participate. This resulted in approximately an additional 75 women coming down to the community center and completing the survey. So this is the strategy that was used when approaching the other PuHDs, especially the large ones. A megaphone was purchased rather cheaply and it was very effective in the beginning to get the women to come down during the day, especially at the time the novellas (Spanish soap opera) are being aired on the local television channels. The research team had already been told that this would probably be a barrier to women's participation. However, the number of women reached in five months suggests it was not a barrier. Overall, this proved the most effective strategy employed to recruit women into the study during the formative phase of the research process. An example of the effectiveness of this strategy lies in the following: over 200 women showed up at Dr. Pila, the largest PuHD here in Ponce, PR. The team actually ran out of questionnaires and had to cut off data collection even though there were still women who wanted to participate. By this time, word had spread throughout the various PuHDs, providing information about the project so that women began to recognize the logo and project name. As such, this resulted in the residents accepting and trusting the project team, and being willing to participate. As a result, data were collected from 1138 women on the quantitative questionnaire. Using the data collected from the quantitative instrument, a qualitative instrument was developed to probe a bit deeper into some of the findings revealed from the analysis of the data set (e.g., their perception of risk, since most women reported being a no risk (approximately 50%)). A convenience sample was used to identify 150 women from various PuHDs, to ensure that there was someone from every PuHD that had been previously visited was included in the sample. As such, all women approached agreed to participate in the face-to-face interview, which took on average between 60 to 120 minutes to complete.

2.3 Obstacles faced during the implementation of *Proyecto MUCHAS*

The project was not without obstacles. The major obstacle faced dealt with the safety issue of the project team performing the research in the PuHDs. However, inner-city, low-income PuHDs are an appropriate and important setting for HIV/STI formative research and subsequent HIV risk reduction interventions. They constitute identifiable and accessible communities in which women at risk for HIV/STI infection can be reached. Characteristics of PuHDs, such as their accessibility, the potential for multiple contacts, and the formulation of resident-controlled intervention components, increase the likely efficacy of such HIV-prevention programs.

This strength, however, is directly related to the major impediment. PuHDs are well-known to have high rates of crime and violence, as well as illicit drug use. Puerto Rico has the highest murder rate in the U.S. and its territories, and 60% of those murders are linked to illegal drugs (Rosa, 2005). The extreme levels of drug-related crime and violence found in PuHDs inevitably contribute to the elevated rates of crime and violence in the overall crime rate in Puerto Rico (Barcelo, 2004). As such, the administration does not allow the research team to go to the residents' apartments and to do the testing and data-collection in private. The team has to go during the day, between the hours of 10:00 a.m. and 7:00 p.m., which are the hours that the administration office is open.

However, the administrative staff has been very helpful, assisting with signing women up and keeping order in the method of data collection, including the testing process. They are also able to identify any person who is not a resident of that specific PuHD but may be trying to participate in the study. As such, this obstacle has weakened the research design, by not allowing the research team to use a random design that was originally proposed. Nevertheless, PuHDs are randomly selected and then every eligible resident is invited to participate. Under the circumstances, this is the best and the strongest design that can be employed, given the realities of the safety issues associated with being in the PuHD.

An example of this concern is illustrated by the following: there were two homicides (both drug-related) that took place last year at the next scheduled site to visit and to conduct HIV/STI testing. Previously, a police officer at this site had expressed his concern for the team's safety and he volunteered to accompany the research team around the complex. This offer was respectfully declined because of concern that it would dissuade participation if team members were accompanied by the police because of fear about informants related to drug use, which is very prevalent in this particular PuHD. Also, associating with the police in front of residents puts the team at increased risk of becoming a victim of drug-related violence.

Overall, residents have been very responsive. The PI had previously conducted some observational research on non-injecting drug use among the residents, to present these data at International Harm Reduction Association Annual Meeting in Warsaw, Poland, in April 2007. During this seven-hour observation, men openly smoked while others bought drugs. Yet, they made the PI feel very comfortable and safe while she was there. One of the men who was there was also a dealer but he trusted the PI to not ''narc'' on him. Unfortunately, he was one of the victims that got shot last year.

This acceptance and trust is vital for the success of a project like this; this also facilitates the willingness of residents' acceptance of and participation in the research project. The residents have been very accepting and trusting, and the team wants to maintain this relationship. Residents recognize the project logo and name and will come down to participate without further use of the megaphone. The team simply puts some posters/flyers up at the mailbox section of the PuHD about a week or two before the site visit, and then when the team arrives, there are many more women waiting to be tested than can be completed in one day. This has been another obstacle faced, along with the realization that we have to work out a way to where we can test the residents in two consecutive days, so they do not get discouraged and are unwilling to come back. However, this issue has to nothing to do directly with the research project but with the disbursement of money from the PI's institution. The research team is currently working with them to resolve this issue.

2.4 Lessons learned from participating in *Proyecto MUCHAS*

Important lessons have been learned during the development and implementation of this project. The most important lesson learned is that it is imperative to treat the residents with respect and not to be judgmental. They respect the team and the team respects them. It was expressed during the focus groups, which were conducted during the formative phase of the research project that they didn't want someone coming over in an "Armani suit" or carrying a "Gucci" handbag trying to talk to them about what it is like to live in a PuHD, because they could not even begin to understand what these residents face and what it is like to be impoverished, with very limited opportunities for betterment (Abreu, et. al., 2010). As such, even if the team is from the Ponce School of Medicine and Health Sciences, it tries to treat them as equals and never pass judgment, even in light of socially undesirable responses (e.g., 95% of the women are unemployed, and only 11% and 22% report using condoms with their last steady and non-steady sex partner) (Norman, et. al., 2010). It is necessary that women feel comfortable enough to share this information, in that these are essential characteristics that keep them in poverty as well as continuing to engage in high risk sexual behaviors. These behaviors include having multiple sex partners, as well as very low rates of condom use reported, and anal intercourse with both steady and non-steady sex partners. In addition, the research team asks about drug use, both a history of and current drug use, which is quite stigmatized, especially among women in PR-- but again, the team does not pass judgment on those who admit a history or current use of illicit drugs, such as heroin and crack-cocaine.

The project team has also learned that these residents want to know more about HIV prevention and strategies to keep them safe. The PuHD administration, based on requests from their residents, has asked the team to prepare and deliver a knowledge and skills-building workshop targeting toward to the PuHD residents to improve knowledge, attitudes, and provide skills in assessing their personal risk of contracting HIV as well as negotiating condom use with their sex partners. This is a positive lesson, in that these women have expressed not only an interest but a desire and willingness to participate in an intervention--if one is developed and implemented targeting them.

In addition, it has been learned that these women have been ignored in previous HIV-related research efforts. As mentioned above, only one study was identified that targeted female residents of public housing and that was almost 20 years ago (Hunt, et. al., 1993). These women are in dire need of HIV prevention interventions, based on their self-reported HIV prevalence rates being over four times of that of the general population of women of the same age group as well as their rates of reported high-risk behaviors. Most HIV-related research has focused on injecting drug use or sex work in and around the San Juan, PR area, especially since injecting drug use is the major mode of HIV transmission among men. However, heterosexual transmission is the major mode among women, constituting approximately two-thirds of all cases (PR Department of Health, 2011). It is an ignominy that no one has recognized the need of these women to receive additional HIV prevention interventions, including continued testing of HIV and other STIs. Residents are highly appreciative of the project and have become very willing to participate. The research team attributes most of the success of this project to date to the participants or residents who live in PuHDs. Without their acceptance of the team and their willingness to participate, the project would not have been able to reach as many women.

3. Recommendations based on our experiences in *Proyecto MUCHAS* and other relevant research

A number of recommendations can be made from the research team's experience with *Proyecto MUCHAS*. The first recommendation would to treat the study population with respect. This is a critical element in implementing a successful HIV-testing outreach project. Related to this recommendation, the researchers should never be judgmental of a participant's responses, even if they do report illegal or socially irresponsible behaviors. It is vital that participants feel comfortable providing these type of sensitive data. A second recommendation is that any potential research project targeting a similar population should be pro-active and aggressive in their recruitment strategies. There are times when traditional recruitment strategies are just not as effective as they need to be. When this happens, a researcher has to be willing to step outside their comfort zone and try something new and innovative, which is what the research team of *Proyecto MUCHAS* did, and it proved to be very successful. And the researchers should never assume that participants are unwilling or uninterested in participating in an intervention, if they believe it will be beneficial to them. However, as mentioned earlier, whomever is chosen to deliver this workshop must be credible but also be accepted and trusted by the participants or they will not trust any information that is being presented to them. The workshop coordinator/presenter must be willing to speak at a level that the participants can understand, as well as show empathy for participants who may be facing extraordinary obstacles to practicing safer sex within their sexual relationships. Also, the team would recommend that each research project develop a logo and a name that participants can associate with the project. The *Proyecto MUCHAS* project developed the logo and name before we ever conducted any data collection (including both the qualitative and quantitative formative data collection). Through the dissemination of information, it will ultimately increase participants' acceptance and willingness to take part in the research project.

4. Implications for future research using this model (*Proyecto MUCHAS*)

There are a number of implications that have arisen from the experience in the development and implementation of *Proyecto MUCHAS.* First, it is important to recognize the vulnerability of public housing residents or low-income and impoverished persons. Research with female public housing residents in the U.S. provides evidence of this vulnerability (Sikemma, 1996; 2000). However, this project focused on prevention of HIV by promoting behavior change. A new paradigm has emerged, which views treatment as a prevention method. This new paradigm, most aggressively led by Julio Montaner, Clinical Director of the BC Centre for Excellence in HIV/AIDS in Vancouver, is frequently referred to as the *Seek-Test-Treat-Retain* strategy (Volkow & Montaner, 2010). The strategy has taken shape as multiple ecological studies emerged, showing the effectiveness of antiretroviral treatment in reducing HIV transmission (Anglemyer, et. al., 2011; Montaner, 2011). In May 2011, results of an NIH-funded trial of this approach known as HPTN 052, filled important gaps in the evidence on efficacy (HIV Prevention Trials Network, 2011). However, it is important to emphasize that HIV treatment is only one of the aspects of HIV prevention efforts that should be targeted toward disadvantaged women. Informing a person of his/her HIV status is the first step. For those who test negative, they are given informational brochures on how to keep from contracting HIV. For those who test positive, we refer them to treatment, along with providing post-test counseling. This post-test counseling includes information on ways they can preventing transmission on to potential sex partners as well as how to protect themselves from re-infections. HIV prevention programs targeting this population must be multi-faceted, including HIV education and skills building, along with HIV testing and following up for treatment for those who test positive.

The result of these developments is that there will be renewed efforts to aggressively implement HIV testing and retention interventions in non-traditional settings (IRIN, 2011). The impetus is not only the need to address significant disparities related to the HIV epidemic, but also the continued lack of substantive progress in the number of people aware of their HIV status, and if positive, linked, and retained into care. Across the most recent studies, approximately one-third to one-half of the newly diagnosed do not connect to care in the post six month period. One in five people who are HIV positive remain unaware of their status in the U.S., with worse estimates for disproportionately affected populations, including those in developing countries (Morin, et. al., 2011). It is important to note that a recent CDC study documented that, similar to the developing world, the U.S. now as a generalized epidemic in urban poverty areas, where four to five times more ethnic minorities reside compared to white (Denning & DiNenno, 2010). However, it is important to recognize that treatment is just one aspect of future HIV transmission. It is to be included in a comprehensive HIV prevention program, first by testing women and informing them of their status. Secondly, HIV prevention information is given to women who test negative but continue to engage in high-risk behaviors. For those that test positive, we refer them to treatment, with treatment now being considered a prevention method for reasons mentioned above. A comprehensive, multi-faceted HIV prevention program is needed for female residents of public housing.

A paradigm of early treatment is still dependent upon early detection, placing even more emphasis on developing innovative strategies of seek and testing and in addressing the acute infection period (Powers, et. al., 20111). However, despite the CDC's nation-wide push to implement routine HIV testing, less than one-third of patents are offered such testing, even where it has been adopted; less than 70% accepted the test (Morin, et. al., 2011).

This is why the success of *Proyecto MUCHAS*, is promising in utilizing a non-traditional setting, removing many obstacles and barriers that persons, especially impoverished minority ones, face. Hopefully, this is just the beginning of an HIV-testing campaign to test all eligible residents of PuHD's in Ponce, PR, and eventually to those in the Southern Region, where approximately 17% of all reported HIV cases exist (Puerto Rico). At this time there are 35,000 residents who live in 73 PuHDs in the Southern region of PR, where Ponce is located, including women and men, adolescents and adults. There is also potential for this study to be replicated in other impoverished communities in PR as well as outside of PR. This model could be applicable with proper cultural adaptation to other countries as well, since subsidized or publicly provided housing is both the norm and highly understudied and underutilized as a venue to HIV prevention.

4.1 HIV engagement or treatment cascade

Another implication is related to the HIV Treatment or Engagement Cascade, which was referred to earlier in the chapter. The strategy of testing and treating as many HIV-positive individuals as possible as a primary prevention strategy has received a great deal of recent attention and advocacy (Dieffenbach CW, Fauci AS, 2009; Granich, et. al., 2009). Universal, voluntary HIV testing has been proposed to identify persons with undetected contracted HIV infection as well as those who are diagnosed but not receiving treatment. Once identified, people diagnosed with HIV should be promptly entered into care and encouraged to initiate and maintain ART regimens to produce viral suppression. In addition to the personal health benefits derived from early HIV identification and treatment, ART that successfully suppresses viral load has been shown to reduce the efficiency of onward disease transmission from infected persons to their sexual partners (Quinn, et. al., 2000; Velasco-Hernandez, Gershengorn HB, Blower SM 2002). Consequently, universal and voluntary HIV testing and antiretroviral treatment of people with HIV is seen as a promising strategy for reducing infectivity and lessening the likelihood of disease transmission (Dieffenbach CW, Fauci AS, 2009; Granich, et. al., 2009). Again, this highlights the importance of testing members of a potentially high-risk of HIV. As such, using *Proyecto MUCHAS* as a model for developing a research project for reaching these impoverished persons may provide the data needed to move HIV-positive participants through the stages of the engagement cascade (Gardner, et. al., 2011). See Figure 3 below for a graphic illustration of the engagement cascade with respect to HIV care.

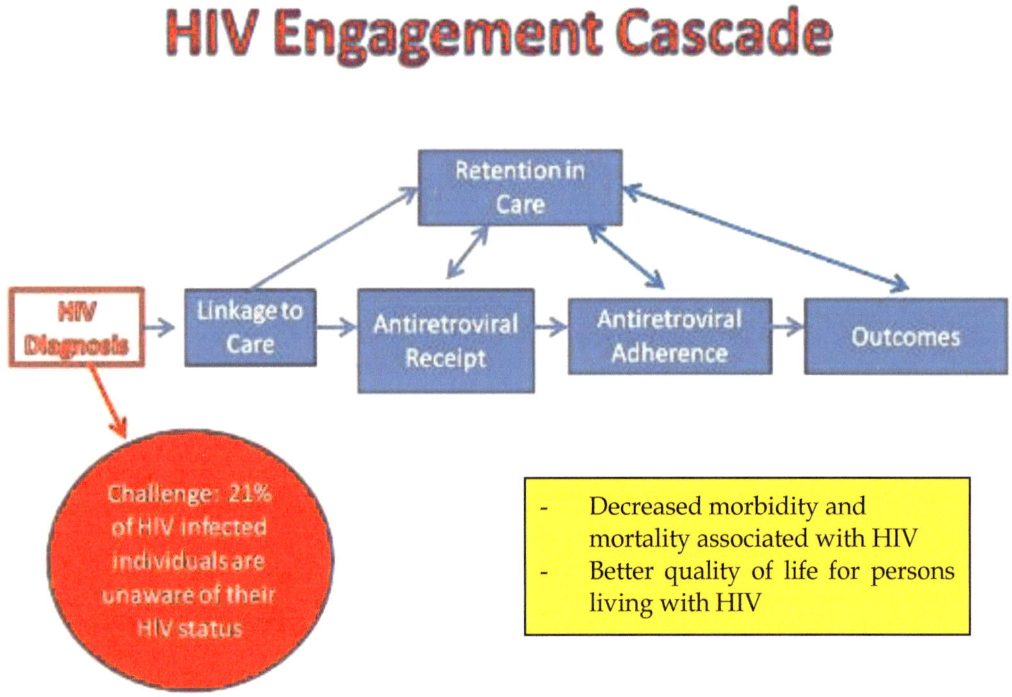

Fig. 3. HIV Engagement Cascade Flowchart

If you notice, HIV testing and diagnosis is highlighted in red, as an indication of its importance in the cascade.

Without HIV testing and informing persons of their status, no further progression can be made with respect to the cascade. HIV testing is the first and can be argued to be the most important step in getting HIV-infected patients linked to and retained in appropriate HIV care and treatment.

5. References

Abreu S, Sala AC, Candelaria EM, Norman LR. (2010). Understanding the barriers that reduce the effectiveness of HIV/AIDS prevention strategies for Puerto Rican women living in low-income households in Ponce, PR: A qualitative study. *Journal of Immigrant and Minority Health*, 2010; 12:83-92.

Antonio-Gaddy M, Richardson-Moore A, Burstein G, Newman D, Branson B, Birkhead G. (2006). Rapid HIV antibody testing in New York State anonymous HIV counseling and testing program. *Journal of Acquired Immune Deficiency Syndromes*, 43, 446-450.

Barcelo, CR. 2004. Crime in Puerto Rico. *Puerto Rico Herald*, July 15.

Brown-Peterside P, Ren L, Chiasson MA, Koblin BA. (2002). Double trouble: violent and non-violent traumas among women at sexual risk of HIV infection. *Women Health*, 36(3):51-64.

Calderon Y, Cowan E, Nickerson J, Mathew S, Fettig J, Rosenberg M, Brusalis C, Chou K, Leider J, Bauman L. (2011). *Pediatrics*, 127, 911-916.

Carovano K. (1992). More than mothers and whores: Redefining the AIDS prevention needs of women. *International Journal of Health Services*, 21(1): 131-142.

Centers for Disease Control and Prevention. (2011). Characteristics associated with HIV infection among heterosexuals in urban areas with high AIDS prevalence --- 24 cities, United States, 2006--2007. *MMWR* ;60:1045-9.

Centers for Disease Control and Prevention. (2010). HIV *Surveillance in Women*. Atlanta, GA: Centers for Disease Control and Prevention.

Centers for Disease Control and Prevention. (2010). *HIV Surveillance Report*. Atlanta, GA: Centers for Disease Control and Prevention.

Centers for Disease Control and Prevention (2008). False-positive oral fluid rapid HIV tests --- New York City, 2005--2008. *MMWR*, 57:1-5.

Centers for Disease Control and Prevention (2007). *Quality Assurance Guidelines for Testing Using Rapid HIV Antibody Tests Waived Under the Clinical Laboratory Improvement Amendments of 1988*. Available at http://www.cdc.gov/hiv/topics/testing/resources/guidelines/pdf/qa_guidlines.pdf.

Centers for Disease Control and Prevention (2007). Rapid HIV testing in emergency departments --- three U.S. sites, January 2005--March 2006. *MMWR*, 56:597-601.

Centers for Disease Control and Prevention. (2006). Revised recommendations for HIV testing of adults, adolescents, and pregnant women in health-care settings. *MMWR Recommendations Report*, 55, 1–17.

Centers for Disease Control and Prevention . (2005). Health disparities experienced by black or African Americans - United States. *MMWR*, 54:1-3.

Centers for Disease Control and Prevention. (2004). *OraQuick Rapid HIV Test for Oral Fluid – Frequently Asked Questions*. Atlanta, GA: Centers for Disease Control and Prevention.

Centers for Disease Control and Prevention. (2003). Advancing HIV prevention: New strategies for a changing epidemic - United States. *MMWR*, 52, 329-332.

Centers for Disease Control and Prevention. (2002). Health-Related Quality of Life --- Puerto Rico, 1996—2000. *MMWR*, 51(08);166-8.

Cichocki, M. (2010). *HIV Timeline - The History of HIV.* Available at http://aids.about.com/od/newlydiagnosed/a/hivtimeline.htm.

Coggins, PC. (2007). *Cultural Issues for HIV/AIDS Clients from the Caribbean: Myths and Realities.* Available at http://www.guyanajpurnal.com/HIV-AIDS_Caribbean.html.

Cohen MS, Chen YQ, McCauley M, Gamble T, Hosseinipour MC Kumarasamy N, ... Fleming TR. (2011). Prevention of HIV-1 Infection with Early Antiretroviral Therapy, *New England Journal of Medicine* l. 365(6): 493-505.

Courtenay, WH. (1998). Better to die than to cry? A longitudinal and constructionist study of masculinity and the health risk behavior of young American men. Doctoral dissertation, University of California, Berkley. Dissertation Abstracts International 59 (08A), Publication number 9902042.

Cummiskey J, Mavinkurve, M, Paneth-Pollak R, Borrelli J. Kowalski A, Blank, S, Branson B. (2008). False-positive oral fluid rapid HIV tests - New York City 2005 - 2008. *MMWR,* 57, 1-5.

Delaney K, Branson B, Uniyal A, Kerndt P, Keenan P, Jafa K, Gardner A, Jamieson D Bulterys M. (2006). Performance of an oral fluid rapid HIV-1/2 test: experience from four CDC studies. *AIDS,* 20, 1655-1660.

Dieffenbach CW, Fauci AS, (2009). Universal voluntary testing and treatment for prevention of HIV transmission. *JAMA,* 301(22): p. 2380-2.

Dinkelman T, Lam D, Leibbrandt M. (2007). Household and community income, economic shocks and risky sexual behavior of young adults: evidence from the Cape Area Panel Study 2002 and 2005. AIDS, 21(Suppl 7):S49-56.

Donnell-Fink L, Reichmann W, Arbelaez C, Case A., Katz J, Losina E, Walensky R. (2011). Patient satisfaction with rapid HIV testing in the emergency department. *Annals of Emergency Medicine,* 58, 49-52.

Fuller CM, Borrell LN, Latkin CA, Galea S, Ompad DC, Strathdee SA, Vlahov D. (2005). Effects of race, neighborhood, and social network on age at indication of injection drug risk. *American Journal of Public Health,* 95(4):689-95.

Galvan F, Bing E, Bluthenthal R., (2000). Accessing HIV Testing and Care. *Journal of Acquired Immune Deficiency Syndromes,* 25, 151-156.

Gardner EM, McLees MP, Steiner JF, Del Rio C, Burman WJ. (2011). The spectrum of engagement in HIV care and its relevant to test-and-treat strategies for prevention HIV infection. *Clinical Infectious Diseases,* 52(6): 793.800.

Granich RM, Gilks CF, Dye C, De Cock KM, Williams BG. (2009). Universal voluntary HIV testing with immediate antiretroviral therapy as a strategy for elimination of HIV transmission: a mathematical model. *Lancet,* 373(9657): p. 48-57.

Greenwald J, Burstein G, Pincus J, Branson B. (2006). A rapid review of rapid HIV antibody tests. *Current Infectious Disease Reports,* 8, 125-131.

Haukoos J, Hopkins E, Hull A, Dean C, Donahoe K, Ruzas C, Bauerie J, Terrien B, Forsyth J, Kalish B, Thrun M, Rothman R. (2011). HIV testing in emergency departments in the United States: A national survey. *Annals of Emergency Medicine,* 58, 10-16.

Henry J. Kaiser Family Foundation. (June, 2005). *HIV Testing in the United States.* Available at http://www.kff.org/hivaids/upload/Updated-Fact-Sheet-HIV-Testing-in-the-United-States.pdf.

Hunt DE, Hammett T, Smith C, Rhodes W, Pares-Avila JA. (1993). Outreach to sexual partners. In Brown BS, Beschner GM (Eds). *Handbook on Risk of AIDS: Injection Drug Users and Sexual Partners.* Westport, Connecticut: Greenwood Press.

Hutchinson A, Farnham P, Lyss S, White D, Sansom, S, Branson B. (2011). Emergency department HIV screening with rapid tests: A cost comparison of alternative models. *AIDS Education and Prevention*, 23, 58-69.

Institute of Medicine. (2011). HIV *Screening and Access to Care: Series Summary.* Available at http://www.iom.edu/2010/HIV-Screening-and Access to Care-Exploring-Barriers.

Johns MM, Bauermeister JA, Zimmerman MA. (2010). Individual and Neighborhood Correlates of HIV testing among African American youth transitioning from adolescence into young adulthood. *AIDS Education and Prevention,* 22(6):509-22.

Kalichman SC, Williams EA, Cherry C, Belcher L, Nachimson D. (1998). Sexual coercion, domestic violence, and negotiating condom use among low-income African American women. *Journal of Women's Health,* 7(3):371-8.

Merchant R, Clark M, Langan T, Mayer K, Seage G, DeGruttola B. (2011). Can computer-based feedback improve emergency department patient uptake of rapid HIV screening? *Annals of Emergency Medicine*, 58, 114-119.

Mesquita F. (April, 2011). Rapid testing - rapid results: Increasing access to HIV testing, results and services. Presenting at World Health Organization Western Pacific Regional Office.

Montaner JSG. (2011). Treatment as prevention—a double hat-trick. *Lancet,* 378:28-209.

Montesinos L, Preciado J. Puerto Rico. In RT Francoeur (Ed.). (2001). The *International Encyclopedia of Sexuality, Volume IV.* New York: The Continuum Publishing Company.

Morin SF, Kelly JA, Charlebois ED, Remien RH, Rotheram-Borus MJ, Cleary PD. (2011). Responding to the national HIV/AIDS strategy-setting the research agenda. *Journal of the Acquired Immune Deficiency Syndrome,* 57(3): 175-80.

Morin S, Khumalo-Sakutukwa G, Charlebois E, Routh J, Fritz K, Lane T, Vaki T, Fiamma A, Coates T. (2006). Removing barriers to knowing HIV status. *Journal of Acquired Immune Deficiency Syndrome,* 41, 218-224.

National Institute of Health. (2011). *HIVAIDS Clinical Trials Network.* Available from http://www.niaid.nih.gov/about/organization/daids/Networks/Pages/daidsnetworks.aspx.

National Minority AIDS Council (2006). *African Americans, Health Disparities and HIV/AIDS: Recommendations for Confronting the Epidemic in Black America.* Washington DC: National Minority AIDS Council.

Norman LR, Abreu S, Candelaria E, & Sala A.(2008). HIV testing practices among women living in public housing in Puerto Rico. *Journal of Women's Health,* 17(4): 641-655.

Norman LR, Abreu S, Candelaria E, Sala A. (2009). The effect of sympathy on discriminatory attitudes toward persons living with HIV/AIDS in Puerto Rico: A hierarchical analysis of women living in public housing. *AIDS Care,* 21(2): 140-149.

Norman LR, Cintron L, Alvarez-Garriga C. (2011). Patterns of condom use among impoverished women living in public housing in Ponce, PR. Oral presentation given at RCMI Annual Meeting, Nashville, TN, December.

Norman LR, Cintron L, Alvarez -Garriga C. (2011). "HIV/STI prevalence among women living in public housing in Ponce, PR. Electronic poster presented at the International AIDS Society Meeting, Rome, Italy, July.

Pacific AIDS Education and Training Center (2009). *Roadmap to Integration: HIV Prevention in Reproductive Health. Tab 8: Conventional and Rapid HIV Testing.* Available at http://www.centerforhealthtraining.org/documents/e09_HIVroadmap.pdf.

Parekh, B., Kalou, M., Alemnji, G., Ou, Chin-Yih, Gershy-Damet, G., and Nkengasong, J. (2010) Scaling up HIV rapid testing in developing countries. *American Journal of Clinical Pathology*, 134, 573-584.

Peltzer, K., Nzewi, E., and Mohan, K. (2004). Attitudes towards HIV-antibody testing and people with aids among university students in India, South Africa and United States. *Indian Journal of Medical Sciences*, 58, 95-108.

Pico I. (1998). *Machismo y Educación.* Rio Piedras: Editorial Universidad de Puerto Rico.

Powers KA, Ghani AC, Miller WC, Hoffman IF, Pettifor AE, Kamanga G, Martinson FE, Cohen MS. (2011). The role of acute and early HIV infection in the spread of HIV and implications for transmission prevention strategies in Lilongwe, Malawi: a modelling study. *Lancet*, 378(9787):256-68.

Prabhu V, Farnham, P, Hutchinson A, Soorapanth S, Heffelfinger J, Golden M, Brooks J, Rimland D, Sansom S. (2011). Cost-effectiveness of HIV screening in STD clinics, emergency departments, and inpatient units: A model-based analysis. *PLoS One*, 6, e19936.

Puerto Rico Department of Health. (2011). *HIV/AIDS Surveillance Report.* San Juan, Puerto Rico: Department of Health.

Quinn TC, et al. (2000). Viral load and heterosexual transmission of human immunodeficiency virus type 1. Rakai Project Study Group. *New England Journal of Medicine*, 342(13): p. 921-9.

Raffaelli M. (2004). Gender socialization in Latino/families: results from two retrospective studies. *Sex Roles: A Journal of Research*, March, 1-24.

Rosa T. (2005). With the highest murder rate in the U.S., Puerto Rico needs immediate solutions. *Puerto Rico Herald*, January 20.

Samet J, Winter M, Grant, L, Hingson R. (1997). Factors associated with HIV testing among sexually active adolescents: A Massachusetts survey. *Pediatrics*, 100, 371-377.

Sanchez T, Sullivan P. (2008). Expanding the horizons: New approaches to providing HIV testing services in the United States. *Public Health Reports*, 123, 1-4.

Scott L, Noble L, Langeveldt M, Jentsch U, Venter F., Daniel W, Stevens W. (2009). Can oral fluid testing be used to replace blood-based HIV rapid testing to improve access to diagnosis in South Africa? *Journal of Acquired Immune Deficiency Syndromes*, 51, 646-648.

Sikemma KJ, Heckman TG, Kelly JA, Anderson ES, Winett RA, Solomon LJ, Wagstaff DA, Roffman RA, Perry MJ, Cargill V, Crumble RW, Fuqua RW, Norman AD, Mercer

MB. (1996). HIV risk behaviors among women living in low-income, inner city housing developments. *American Journal of Public Health,* 86(8):1123-8.

Sikemma, KJ, Kelly JA, Winett RA, Solomon LJ, CA., MD, Roffman RA, McAuliffe TL., Heckman TG., Anderson EA ,

Simon PA, Hu DJ, Diaz T, Kerndt PR. (1995). Income and AIDS rates in Los Angeles County. *AIDS,* 9(3):281-4.

Spielberg F, Branson B, Goldbaum G, Lockhart, D, Kurth A, Celum C, Rossini A, Critchlow C, Wood R.. (2003). Overcoming barriers to HIV testing: Preferences for new strategies among clients of a needle exchange, a sexually transmitted disease clinic, and sex venues for men who have sex with men. *Journal of Acquired Immune Deficiency Syndromes,* 32, 318-327.

Spielberg F, Branson B, Goldbaum G, Lockhart D, Kurth A, Rossini, A, Wood R.. (2005). Choosing HIV counseling and testing strategies for outreach settings: A randomized trial. *Journal of Acquired Immune Deficiency Syndromes,* 38, 348-355.

Steele C, Meléndez-Morales L, Campoluci R, DeLuca N, Dean H. (2007). *Health Disparities in HIV/AIDS, Viral Hepatitis, Sexually Transmitted Diseases, and Tuberculosis: Issues, Burden, and Response: A Retrospective Review, 2000–2004. Atlanta, GA: Department of Health and Human Services, Centers for Disease Control and Prevention.* Available at: http://www.cdc.gov/nchhstp/healthdisparities/.

Sudley B, Stith A, Nelson A. (2002). *Unequal Treatment: Confronting Racial and Ethnic Disparities in Health Care.* Washington DC: National Academies Press.

U.S. Department of Health and Human Services. (2011). *HIV.* Available at http://www.healthypeople.gov/2020/topicsobjectives2020/overview.aspx?topicid=22.

U.S. Department of Health and Human Services. (2011). *Secretary's Advisory Committee on National Health Promotion and Disease Prevention Objectives for 2020.* Available at:

U.S. Census Bureau. (2011). *United States Census 2010.* Washington, D.C.: U.S. Census Bureau, Public Information Office.

Van Griensven, F. (2011). *HIV Rapid Testing: Experiences from the Silom Community Clinic, 2005 - 2011.* Available from http://www.aidstar onc.com/sites/default/files/technical_consultations/rapid_testing_rapid_results/day_1/Frits_van_Griensven.pdf..

Velasco-Hernandez JX, Gershengorn HB, Blower SM. (2002). Could widespread use of combination antiretroviral therapy eradicate HIV epidemics? *Lancet Infectious Diseases,* 2(8): p. 487-93.

Viall A, Dooley S, Branson B, Duffy N, Mermin J, Cleveland J, Cagle C, Lyon W. (2011). Results of the expanded HIV testing initiative - 25 jurisdictions, United States, 2007-2010. *MMWR,* 60, 805-810.

Volkow ND, Montaner J. (2010). Enhanced HIV Testing, Treatment, and Support for HIV-Infected Substance Users. *Journal of the American Medical Association,* 303(14):1423-1424.

Wagstaff DA, Norman AD. Perry MJ, Crumble DA, Mercer MB. *(2000).* Outcomes of a randomized community-level HIV prevention intervention for women living in 18 low-income housing developments. *American Journal of Public Health,* 90(1):57-63.

Women's Health. (2011). Women and HIV/AIDS. Available at http://www.womenshealth.gov/hiv-aids/women-are-at-risk-of-hiv/

5

Perceptions About Barriers and Promoting Factors Among Service Providers and Community Members on PMTCT Services

Fyson H. Kasenga
Malawi Union of Seventh Day Adventist church, Health Ministries Department, Malawi

1. Introduction

Mother-to-child transmission (MTCT) of HIV is a global problem. Annually, MTCT accounts for almost two-thirds of the new infections that occur in children world-wide. Each year, at least 2 million women become infected with HIV, mainly as a result of heterosexual transmission, and approximately 750 000 children acquire HIV infection, mostly through MTCT. MTCT varies widely and is dependent on obstetric practices, mode of delivery, breastfeeding, and the mother's level of the viral load. (Moodley and Moodley 2005; UNAIDS, 2004). HIV is transmitted from mother-to-child at various stages of pregnancy including in utero, intrapartum and during breastfeeding. Untreated 20-40% of infants born to HIV infected mothers will be infected as well, whereas a combination of antiretroviral therapy during pregnancy, elective caesarean section and bottle feeding reduce the risk of vertical transmission to below 2% (Newell, 2006).

There are over 42 million people living with HIV/AIDS worldwide, 38.6 million of these are adults, 19.2 million are women and 3.2 million are children aged below 15. A total of over 3 million people have already died of HIV/AIDS related illness. More than 90% of people living with HIV are in developing countries, with sub-Saharan Africa accounting for two thirds of all the HIV-infected people in the world (AMN, 2005; UNAIDS, 2004). As the virus is predominantly transmitted through sexual contact, equal numbers of males and females are infected, mainly young people of reproductive age. Hence, there is a growing number of HIV positive children infected during pregnancy, delivery or through breast milk. The interventions have therefore, been aimed at effectively providing alternatives to breastfeeding and limiting the risk of newborn infection. Some of the interventions that limit MTCT are using caesarian section as the mode of delivery and administering antiretroviral (ARV) drugs prepartum and peripartum. However, these approaches are not always possible in developing countries and the use of ARV drugs, in particular nevirapine (NVP), zidovudine (ZDV) and zidovudine/lamivudine, have been investigated in both developing and developed countries (Giaquito et al., 2006). Although the available methods of interventions are widely used in the industrialized world, implementation seems difficult in developing countries because of political, financial, logical and societal factors. Screening of pregnant women and identification of HIV positive mothers can result in violence, rejection and stigmatization, and has to be put in the balance of programmes aiming at reducing the number of infected children.

Malawi's HIV infection rate is estimated to be at least 14% among the adult population aged between 15 - 49 (MDHS, 2004). Over 70% of hospital beds in Malawi are occupied by people with HIV/AIDS related conditions. Survey of tuberculosis (TB) patients has revealed that over 70% are co-infected with HIV. Life expectancy which was estimated to have been over 55 years without AIDS has now come down to 42 for men and 41 for women with AIDS (UNAIDS 2006). Of the people infected with HIV virus, women and children are more infected than men. It is estimated that HIV prevalence among pregnant women may be between 19 and 30 percent (Baylor aids, 2005).

PMTCT programmes continue to be a priority as MTCT accounts for 30 percent of all new infections in Malawi and is the second major mode of transmission after unprotected sex. Every year, an estimated 30,000 babies are born HIV positive. It was for this reason that in 2001, Malawi initiated 3 PMTCT sites and in 2003, the launching was done. PMTCT programmes are being implemented by every district in Malawi and by end of 2005, PMTCT services were being implemented in 36 sites (Buhendwa, 2003). Relatively simple interventions to lower the risk of infection are available to only a small number of women and lag far behind the country's antiretroviral therapy (ART) programme, which now reaches 70,000 HIV-infected people or about 40 percent of those who need them. In 2005, 5,054 women received NVP, an ARV drug that lowers the chances of a mother infecting her baby by up to 40 percent. This was almost twice the number who received the drug in 2004 but in reality there is less total number of pregnant women in Malawi who accessed PMTCT services so far as more pregnant mothers continue to be infected (IRIN, 2007).

With the introduction of opt-out strategy in the PMTCT programme, most antenatal mothers fail to access the services as required due to problems. Women feared transportation and supplementary food costs, referral hospitals' reputation for being unfriendly and confusing and difficulties in sustaining long-term treatment would limit accessibility. Fear of stigma framed all concerns, posing challenges for contacting referrals who did not want their status disclosed (Mshana et al., 2006). The problems that limit women to access the PMTCT services can be minimized if they hold dialogue with their spouses before HIV testing. This is because as they accept HIV testing, some women decide not to inform their spouses when tested in the absence of the male spouse. Male involvement and couple counseling have been advocated as having a positive influence on the women's accessibility to the PMTCT services (Homsy et al., 2006).

A single dose of NVP given to the mother at the onset of labour and to the baby within 72 hours after delivery reduces HIV transmission rates by 38-50% and is relatively cheap and easy to administer (Avert.org. 2005; Lallemant et al., 2004; Halkin *et al.,* 2005, Scarlatti, 2004). While this is an opportunity to provide infected mothers with the ART, there is also need for mothers to know and accept their situation.

Not all antenatal mothers in the Malamulo Hospital catchment area access maternal services at the hospital. Some of them continue to access delivery services at the traditional birth attendants (TBAs) despite attending antenatal services. More emphasis is put on the women to understand their situation and access PMTCT services but PMTCT coverage continues to be low. Not much is reported about the perceptions and factors of the service providers and communities hindering antenatal mothers from accessing PMTCT services. Therefore, the study aimed at exploring barriers and promoting factors to delivery of PMTCT services as perceived by service providers and community members. The findings would be useful in providing the basis for understanding women's situations and be able to provide them with the needed support in order to increase accessibility of PMTCT services and reduce MTCT.

2. Methods

2.1 Study design

Qualitative study using focus group discussions (FGDs), part of wider operations of HIV/AIDS prevention project around local introduction and scale up of PMTCT services for antenatal mothers.

2.2 Study area

Malamulo mission hospital is owned by the Seventh Day Adventist Church and is located in the southern region of Malawi, 65 km south east of Blantyre City in Thyolo District. It was established in 1902 and remains the headquarters of the Adventist Church in Malawi. The hospital has 15 mobile sites with 2 health centres and collaborates with other Non-Governmental Organizations (NGOs) including Thyolo District Hospital. The Government and NGOs deliver health care in Malawi. Among the NGOs, faith based institutions ran health facilities but are subsidized by the Government. These faith based health facilities belong to an organization called Christian Health Association of Malawi (CHAM). Malamulo hospital has a membership to this organization and the study was done within its catchment area.

Malamulo runs an Integrated HIV/AIDS Prevention Project with local and external support. At the time when this study was done, it was largely funded by USAID through an international organization called Private Partners Collaborating Together (PACT). The components were voluntary counseling and testing (VCT), management of sexually transmitted infections (STIs), home based care (HBC), youth friendly health services (YFHS), family planning (FP), prevention of mother to child transmission (PMTCT) of HIV, ART provision, nutrition, static and outreach mother and child health (MCH) services.

Thyolo is one of the districts in Malawi that receives highest rainfall annually. Tea and coffee estates surround Malamulo hospital. The hospital is one of the teaching institutions in the country for allied health workers and has 300 beds. It serves an estimated population of a little over 70,000. Communication is a problem due to poor roads and worsens during rainy season. The people's socio-economic status in this area is low. Many of them are seasonal migrant workers for the tea and coffee estates. Most people are peasant farmers who grow maize, beans, cassava and bananas mainly for home consumption. Crop harvest is usually poor since most of the people are not using modern farming methods. Malnutrition, communicable diseases such as malaria, worm infestation, TB, diarrhea diseases and STIs including HIV/AIDS are common. HIV prevalence in this population is 16% slightly higher than the national one of 14% (MDHS, 2004). Many families have experienced a loss of a member due to AIDS and the number of orphans is also high. Cultural practices such as wife inheritance among other factors are responsible for HIV proliferation.

2.3 Malamulo hospital PMTCT Programme

Malamulo hospital PMTCT services began in July 2004. More antenatal care (ANC) mothers accessing services at Malamulo tested HIV positive. Malawi Government through its Health Ministry assessed the hospital and determined it legible for the ART provision in the area. Malamulo began full ART service provision in August 2004. Over 500 people have already accessed ART, 200 HIV infected antenatal mothers and 100 babies have been provided with NVP.

Malamulo PMTCT programme is a PMTCT plus because it supports the provision of specialised care to HIV-infected women namely ART, STIs, HBC, infant feeding practices and nutrition. It further adopts national and international standards according to World Health Organisation (WHO). The strategies used are primary prevention in child bearing age for both men and women, prevention of unwanted pregnancy, prevention of HIV infection from an infected mother to the child by providing NVP to them, counsel and support on safe infant feeding, care continuum for mother and baby. The working areas are antenatal, labour and delivery, postnatal and community support.

2.4 Sampling of informants

The informants were purposively selected based on the theoretical assumption that there were variations and range of perceptions by community members and service providers towards the delivery of Malamulo Hospital PMTCT services. The informants were in five groups namely: 1) men, 2) women, 3) village headmen, 4) religious leaders and 5) health workers. These were community members from the 15 villages that surround the hospital and were in their child bearing ages and beyond. Their proximity to the hospital, involvement in the health services and being within 15 villages from where most service users come including antenatal mothers made them legible to participate in the study. On average, participants lived at distance ranging from 5 - 15 km away from the hospital and for logistic reasons; it was possible to reach them at such a distance.

2.5 Data collection

The audio taped FGDs were conducted from October 2006 - February 2007. Appointments to get permission to conduct FGDs were made to the village headmen, heads of household and the participants before the due dates. At the time of appointments, explanations were made about who the researcher was, the fact that the study would help to get deeper understanding of their perceptions about barriers and promoting factors on the delivery of PMTCT services and possible benefits. A guide was used during the FGDs in an open conversation. It consisted of themes namely; role in pregnancy and sickness, common practices and norms related to pregnancy, home or hospital deliveries, antenatal and PMTCT services. One FGD was postponed to a later date because it was raining heavily and there was a function at the venue on that day.

Two pictures showing hospital and home deliveries were used as a starter. A total of 9 FGDs were conducted by the author with two assistants. Of these, 2 sessions were held with each of the following; women, men, village headmen, religious leaders and 1 with the health workers. To ensure privacy, all FGDs were done in a room as per participants' choice. The local school head master permitted us to use one of his school classrooms. Participants anonymously agreed to start the discussions and end with prayers. The discussions were conducted in the afternoon to accommodate the working schedules of the participants. As no new information seemed to be emerging, and given the paucity of the participants who were willing to share openly about their perceptions towards PMTCT services, data collection was deemed complete after the ninth group. The FGDs lasted from 90 to 135 minutes. Participants were served with soft drinks before returning to their homes.

2.6 Data analysis

Data were analyzed qualitatively using content analysis guided by Graneheim and Lundman (2004). The process was facilitated by use of the open code soft ware developed at Umeå University, Sweden (Open Code, 2007). Texts were transcribed verbatim, open coding, categories, properties and dimensions were made (Tables 1, 2 and 3). Based on the coded data and themes were developed to explain perceptions about barriers and promoting factors among service providers and community members on the delivery of the PMTCT services.

2.7 Ethical consideration

Consent was obtained from Malamulo Hospital Administrative Council. Chiefs and respondents gave their oral informed consent as well. A further permission was obtained from the Health Sciences Research Council in the Ministry of Health, Malawi. All the respondents were assured that information given would be treated with strict confidentiality.

Extra marital sex	Self decided	Delivered alone	Unfaithful
Sex abstinence	Partner involvement	Disappointing	HIV testing
Pregnancy	ANC information	Women shouted	Prevention
Norms	Money given	No attention	Protective
Love	Husband prepared	Good	Infected women
Sex life	Hospital	Kind	Unprotected
Marriage	Delivery	Respect	Sickness
Stillbirth	Home	Uninterested	Condom use
Shameful	Timing	Abandon	Counseled
Adultery	Relatives involved	Patients	Cried for self
Church beliefs	Support	Problem	Health workers

Table 1. List of open codes

Beliefs	HIV testing	Place of delivery	Role in sickness and pregnancy	Suggested solutions
Couples counseled	Condom use	No medicine at home	Supportive man	Promote condom use
Couples to be faithful	Unfaithful man	Unskilled TBAs	Prayed for sickness	H/workers as models
Sex stops before delivery	Infected couples	TBAs are attentive	Sick sent to hospital	Team work
Sex resumes after delivery	Tested HIV positive	Less expensive care	Preparations made	Older nurses to help
Herbs used in pregnancy	Wife took HIV test	Safe hospital delivery	Child care	Leadership to help
Fisi allowed if man infertile	Husband refused	Distance, sudden pains	Pregnant lady to rest	Educate communities
Baby covered with sperms	STIs are dangerous	Abandoned women	Husband to love wife	Less trainees in ward
Sex nourishes pregnancy	Protection	Women deliver alone	Church helps in kind	Behavioral change
Never eat eggs in pregnancy	ART-benefits	Decision discussed	Chiefs help the sick	Empower community
Offals uneaten in pregnancy	Babies free of HIV	Decision made alone	Patients' care	Discuss problems
Socks not used in pregnancy				

Table 2. Categories

Category	Properties	Dimensions
Discrimination	Extent	Less or more
Few months	Extent	Less or more
Behavioral change	Degree	Self or others
Disease	Degree	Self or others
Support	Origin	Felt or enacted
Responsibility	Origin	Felt or enacted
Environment	Impact	Partly or fully

Table 3. Examples of categories, properties and dimensions

3. Results

A total of 9 FGDs were conducted with 69 participants grouped by gender, age and occupation. At least one member from the 15 villages that surround the hospital participated in the discussions. Of the 69 participants, 47 were males and 22 were females with the mean age of 28.5 years. Fifty six were married and thirteen were singles. The participants' number of children ranged from 1 to 8 with average to low socio-economic status. The clergy represented Christians and Moslems and so were the participants. The participants' education ranged from primary school to tertiary levels and five had none.

Four themes about barriers and promoting factors on PMTCT services as perceived by service providers and community members emerged: 1) Decision: Place of delivery, 2) Perceptions concerning service providers at hospital and home deliveries, 3) Perceptions of the role of communities during pregnancy and sickness and 4) Perceptions of community interventions (Table 4). Decision: Place of delivery was referred to the decision maker and the circumstances that surrounded the place of choice for delivery. Perceptions concerning service providers at hospital and home deliveries was referred to the attitude and knowledge of the birth attendants at community and hospital levels.

Perceptions of the role of communities during pregnancy and sickness referred to the responsibilities assumed by communities at different levels in taking care of pregnant women and the sick. Perceptions of community interventions referred to suggested solutions to improve service delivery and accessibility as perceived by the participants. Involvement of care givers and their recipients is included in this theme.

3.1 Decision: Place of delivery

Men decided for their pregnant wives where to deliver and to a large extent women obeyed their husbands' decisions. Some informants reported that decisions were discussed between partners, partners and family members and in certain rare situations women decided by themselves. Grandmothers, mothers and friends influenced the decisions based on their past delivery experiences. It was mentioned that previous experiences with the health facilities such as ANC information, treatment in the ANC and labour ward and family support influenced decisions about where to deliver. A female participant explained how her husband decided for her where to deliver:

"For me it is my husband who reminds me when to begin ANC. This is because he knows my dates and is very good at encouraging me to go for hospital delivery. He also keeps money to meet delivery expenses. He buys me a piece of cloth, basin and a plastic bag among other things".

Codes	Categories	Themes
My decision Husband's decision Discussed with partner Mother's decision Grandmother's decision Relative's decision Friends' decision Useful ANC information Given money by husband Husband-encouraging Safe hospital delivery Unsafe home delivery	Supportive husband Family support Supportive health care system Tradition	Decision: Place of delivery
Rude nurses in labour ward Delivered alone in labour ward Female nurses -disrespecting Male nurses- helpful Polite nurses in ANC Women respected in ANC Trainee nurses-less competent Trainee nurses-playful Hospital skilled personnel Home-unskilled personnel TBAs respect women TBAs' care is good	Health workers' supportive attitude Health workers' unsupportive attitude Health workers' job knowledge	Perceptions concerning service providers at hospital and home deliveries
Prepared for delivery experiences Material and moral support Couples advised on norms to follow TBAs-important for delivery Traditional healers-important for sickness Home remedy-priority before hospital Hospital treatment-encouraged Spiritual support Communities' help Patients' visited HIV/AIDS awareness Circumstances	Family care Community care Religious perspective Health personnel's views	Perceptions of the role of communities during pregnancy and sickness
Trainees supervised Health promotion Labour ward-full time nurse Leadership-important Approachable male nurses Behavioural change Promote condom use Women' early reporting Good nurses rewarded Rude nurses reprimanded Trained TBAs- important Traditional norms complied	Interventions at hospital level Interventions at community level Service recipients' role	Perceptions of community interventions

Table 4. Themes, categories and codes

Participants reported that hospital delivery was better because of safety as opposed to home delivery. Some participants felt that although home delivery was regarded as unsafe but was ideal for them because they got used to certain birth attendants and needed no preparations to access the services. It was further cited by one male participant whose wife had 8 home deliveries without complications that it was relatively cheap to have home delivery as compared with hospital delivery.

Participants stated that complications with home deliveries such as maternal and child deaths influenced women to seek hospital deliveries. Female participants with past hospital and home delivery experiences described home delivery area as unhygienic which would predispose them to infection after delivery and such situation rarely happened with hospital delivery. Participants' views on where to deliver were explained in the following way:

"Women deliver at home because of negligence, beliefs and lack of transport. They say if grandmothers had several home deliveries without complications, why bother and have specific people to assist them during delivery. Home delivery women with difficulties seek hospital deliveries and these are good examples for women in the communities to appreciate the hospital services".

3.2 Perceptions concerning service providers at hospital and home deliveries

Female participants reported that nurses in the ANC were kind, polite and willing to help and male participants had similar impressions from their wives. Nurses in the ANC provided the women with adequate information on various health issues, treated women with respect, and motivated them to attend ANC. It was also mentioned that traditional birth attendants were equally good at treating women with care and respect and this attracted more women to them.

Participants reported that nurses in the labour ward did not respect them, were rude, and shouted at women during delivery and some of them delivered alone. This situation made women have their deliveries at the traditional birth attendants where respect and kindness were shown to them regardless of regular ANC attendance. Below is the description on how participants viewed service providers at ANC and labour ward:

"The antenatal care clinic is fine but difficulties are found in labour ward. As nurses conduct examinations in the labour ward, the way they talk it is as if they are not willing to help. In the antenatal care, we are free to ask questions and the nurses explain and answer most of them and wherever necessary, we are referred to a doctor depending on our problems".

Some participants expressed that male nurses were kind, respected them during delivery and were full time in labour ward monitoring the women until delivery:

"Female nurses are rude in the labour ward. They often tell pregnant woman that her time for delivery is not yet due while it is not true. As the woman leaves the labour ward she delivers on her own. My wife told me and this happened to her. Male nurses behave well and assist women to deliver with respect, dignity and rarely women complain of them".

All the participants stated that service providers at the hospital had knowledge, skills, medications and equipment to carry out their functions in a professional way. Therefore, they felt that hospital delivery was safe because if something went wrong during delivery, women would easily be assisted. It was mentioned that birth attendants at home had little or no education, limited knowledge, skills and lacked equipment to carry out the delivery services. Some participants stated that it was mere chance that women had successful home deliveries and recalled several incidences where women or infants died during delivery. They said that women die from preventable causes from home delivery.

3.3 Perceptions of the role of communities during pregnancy and sickness

All the participants stated that pregnancy needed their attention to enable women deliver successfully. Couples had sole responsibilities for the care and particularly the husband was expected to look after his pregnant wife as determined by marriage counsels. It was mentioned that during pregnancy, the couples were advised to follow the norms and make preparations for deliveries. At family level the pregnant woman was provided with basic needs such as food and was advised to start ANC on time. Participants viewed both pregnancy and sickness as events that brought all the communities together. Below is the participants' common impression on sickness:

"I take part in pregnancy and sickness. When one of my family members gets sick, I send him to the hospital for treatment. I do the same with anyone within my village. We use a stretcher to carry the sick to the hospital. We often come together as people living in the village to help carry the sick to the hospital. We do not leave this task with the patients' families only".

People outside the families helped pregnant women especially if their families were failing to fulfill certain obligations such as encouraging early antenatal attendance and material support. The religious leaders provided the pregnant women with moral and spiritual support and the participants encouraged utilization of heath services during pregnancy and sickness. Health personnel participants stated that some young women failed to attend ANC because of laziness and obedience to their older women who usually encouraged home delivery. They further said that they were eager to see as many women in the ANC and delivery suits as possible to reduce maternal and infants mortality rates.

It was mentioned that pregnancy and sickness were associated with norms and traditional healers or birth attendants were consulted before going to the hospital. Some traditional beliefs encouraged regular intake of local herbs, home delivery and discouraged antenatal attendants to avoid getting instructions which were difficult to follow. Pregnant women were disallowed to eat offals, stand or sit at the door and husbands were not allowed to put on neck ties or socks because such things would lead to difficulties in delivery. They were further discouraged from eating eggs because this would cause chronic abdominal pains. Coincidentally, one of the HIV infected participants shared his experiences with others in stressing the importance of seeking medical treatment in sickness in the following way:

"I got sick for a long time, eaten several herbs but did not help me until the time I went to the hospital. I tested HIV positive and I do not hide, I tell people about this. I tell them that if they fall sick, they should go to the hospital. If I did not go to the hospital, by now I should have been dead. Today I have life and leading the normal life. I am the living example and I tell people in my village to first go to the hospital. If there is no improvement after going to the hospital, then they can go to the traditional healers".

On average, the participants abstained from sexual contact between 6-8 months before delivery and resumed it 6 months after delivery. They followed this norm to avoid traumatizing the infants, delivering deformed babies covered with sperms, malnutrition or having unwanted pregnancies. It was also reported that participants were advised to stick to each other if they were married and HIV negative (practice mutual faithfulness), use condoms if they were HIV positive or not sure of their HIV status or practice abstinence if they were not married to avoid contracting sexually transmitted infections and HIV/AIDS. Where men failed to have their wives pregnant, elders arranged that fertile men slept with the women on mutual agreements with their husbands. The practice was called **"Fisi"** but was being discouraged nowadays due to HIV/AIDS.

The participants expected women to be submissive to their husbands in all matters relating to family life. Male participants suggested that before going for HIV testing, women should consult their husbands as failure to do so would cause family problems. Some participants felt that they would go for HIV testing if they thought of being HIV infected or if they got sick.

3.4 Perceptions of community interventions

While participants mentioned the health systems' strengths and weaknesses, also chanted the way forward. Some participants reported that the improvements should involve all the partners who came into play. They mentioned that the health facility's leadership should help the service providers' attitudinal change into a more responsive and willingness to care for the recipients. The participants suggested the following; health promotion, trainee supervision, rewarding hard working nurses, disciplining the rude nurses and communicating the effected changes with the communities. All participants mentioned that the labour ward needed much attention as other hospital departments. Participants felt that it was the right time to express their problems:

"The problem is with us because we hide. When the woman is in labour, the nurses are usually not present. The woman delivers alone and this is the report that we often get. Here we need to correct the situation. We request that nurses should be able to monitor the woman who goes into labour until delivery".

The ages of the trainee nurses and how they handled women in labour ward raised concerns:

"The problem is that some of the nurses are very young, never delivered before but have to conduct deliveries. They disrespect the pregnant mothers due to lack of experience. It is important that a qualified nurse should always guide trainee nurses so that what is done should be of high quality and standard".

The participants requested training of the traditional birth attendants (TBAs) to assist women who may access their services due to unavoidable circumstances such as sudden labour pains. Some participants felt that empowerment of local communities would help them to be responsible for their health issues. Participants reported that individual families and the women should understand the importance of accessing health care services on time. It was mentioned that early reporting in sickness and regular ANC attendance, hospital delivery and discouraging norms that were detrimental to their health would be the way forward.

All participants were responsible for the sick in their communities and needed them to access health facility treatment on time. They further reported that they discouraged the tendency of seeking traditional remedy before the modern medical treatment. Health personnel participants felt that they needed to be role models and be able to treat their service users with respect and dignity. Below is their expression on this:

"We need to be role models. Pregnant women should be given time to explain their side of the story and do as they wish. They should be told properly about HIV testing and allowed to decide to take the test or not. They should never be shouted at since pregnancy and delivery are stressful".

4. Discussions

The study revealed that men largely decided for their pregnant wives where to access health care and delivery services. This is consistent with the conversional wisdom that men are dominant decision makers in matters relating to fertility (Maharaj and Cleland, 2005). This has several implications; it may be a male dominant society where men are decision makers for their families leading to women's limitations in making independent choices for their lives as is the case in other societies (Santelli et al, 2006). Further, if men were unsupportive then their wives may be negatively affected and in certain situations, family support, positive health care reputations and discussions with wives influenced decisions. Women verified their decisions with husbands, relatives or friends and were inclined to seek home delivery which showed that traditional beliefs were deep rooted in this society. This may also suggest that women in this study were less empowered to pose as powerful predictor of where they would wish to deliver.

The study showed that service providers at health facility and local levels influenced the community's acceptability and accessibility of the health services including PMTCT services. This is an important finding and it may imply that utilization of the health service is dependent on how well the recipients are treated, the trust the service users have in the service providers and the job knowledge. However, attitude and ability to treat patients with dignity and respect have a great role in influencing people's willingness to access the services (Mathole et al., 2005; Owens, 2005; Hilget and Gill, 2007). This may suggest that people seek traditional health care than modern health so long they feel welcomed and seen not as nuisance preventing others from resting. Interestingly, male nurses were more preferred than female nurses by women in the labour ward because of their dedication and respect they showed to the women in caring for them to deliver. This further implies that the long traditional culture that disregarded male nurses in delivery places is changing. Males are therefore equally accepted to conduct deliveries in labour ward as female nurses given the job knowledge and eagerness to utilize it in a dignified manner.

Pregnancy and sickness in general seemed to be community unifying events in this study. Families and communities at various levels took part in alleviating human suffering. This is congruent with what was obtained before (Mant et. al., 2005). This has several implications; families prepared for pregnant outcome and this extend to the community at large where responsible individuals were indoctrinated with traditional ideologies coupled with modern health care. Primarily, pregnant women and the sick sought remedies for their ailments from the traditional birth attendants or traditional healers and if encountered no problems, it became the habit at the expense of the modern health care. This suggests an opportunity to instill long lasting modern health care messages which are likely to be well taken up as is the case with traditional beliefs provided the messages are linked with live examples of health benefits. Communities followed traditional norms that had no health benefits and to some were detrimental to their health (Banda et al., 2007; Kamatenesi-Mugisha and Oryem-Origa, 2006). Interestingly, customs such as wife inheritance and temporal allowance of fertile men to sleep with women whose men were infertile through mutual agreement is dying away due to HIV/AIDS. This is an indication that communities understand the dangers HIV/AIDS inflicts upon them, hence take active roles in fighting against HIV/AIDS.

The study has revealed that the interventions deemed important for the acceptability, affordability and accessibility of the services by women as well as the community at large.

This concurs with what was found before that community involvement and participation are known as key elements in any given successful community projects (Loss et al., 2007; Bhuyan, 2004). This may be explained in that the communities see the project as "our project" and not "their project". The health facility's leadership needed to look into its staffing problems particularly in labour ward where women complained of the nurses. This implies that the hospital needs to intensify its service delivery strategies, by hiring competent and dedicated health workers or motivating the existing members of staff to do the right thing for the women and the sick at large. However, the changes made at the hospital should contain improved communication of the services provided to the community.

The community's willingness to step up their efforts in utilizing health care services seems to be dependent on their relationship with the health service providers and the understanding health implications. This implies that there should be a trigular type of relationship involving the service providers at community and health facility levels and the communities themselves. It was evident in this study that various stakeholders experienced weaknesses in themselves and health workers in particular, pledged to be role models and would give a different face value in their health delivery involvement. This suggests that there was a reflection of what actually happens in each of the key players and there is a possibility of a change for the better.

It was further revealed that women should consult their husbands before undergoing HIV testing. This is important in that the adoption of such practice would spare women from experiencing problems within their families and has been supported by studies before (Kakimoto et al., 2007; Homsy et al., 2006). This implies that women would not fear disclosing their HIV status hence not bullied or beaten up by their husbands and can pave ways for more men to access HIV testing. This may as well facilitate family unification and creation of positive living within couples' relationships while living with HIV/AIDS.

Financial constraints, author's hospital representation and distance to find the study participants were the study limitations. The study has the strength of exploring barriers and promoting factors to delivery of PMTCT services as perceived by service providers and community members. Further, inclusion of participants at various levels poses a fair representation of the study findings useful for service delivery improvements.

Men were decision makers in matters relating to pregnancy and where their wives should deliver, service providers' attitude and knowledge affected health care service delivery, pregnancy and sickness were seen as unifying events by the communities. Improved communication between service providers and service users were the suggested intervention measures. Based on these findings, we recommend training of the TBAs and women's empowerment to make independent choices in matters relating to pregnancy and child births.

5. Acknowledgement

We thank the Swedish Institute, Sweden for the financial support without which the study would have been a non starter. We are also grateful for the support given by the unit of Epidemiology and Public Health Sciences, Umeå University. Furthermore, we thank the management and staff of Malamulo SDA Hospital, P/Bag 2, Makwasa and Malawi Union of

SDA Church, Malawi for their support throughout the entire period of carrying out this piece of work.

6. References

Armenian Medical Network (AMN). (2005). HIV/AIDS, HIV and the Acquired Immunodeficiency Syndrome, HIV/AIDS Health Centre

UNAIDS. (2004). Report on the global AIDS epidemic, Geneva.

AVERT.Org, (2004). Starting Antiviral Treatment, *Averting HIV/AIDS.Org.*

Banda Y, Chapman V, Goldenberg RL, Stringer JS, Culhane JF, Sinkala M, Vermund SH, Chi BH. (2007). Use of traditional medicine among pregnant women in Lusaka, Zambia, Journal of Alternative and Complementary Medicine, 13(1):123-7.

Bhuyan KK. (2004). Health promotion through self-care and community participation: elements of a proposed programme in the developing countries, BMC Public Health, 4: 11.

Baylor aids (2005). BIPAI programmes: Malawi, Facts on HIV/AIDS in Malawi, *Baylor international Pediatrics AIDS Initiative, Bayloraids.Org.*

Buhendwa L. (2003). PMTCT services in Malawi. Medicins Sans frontiers (MSF/B), Malawi.

Giaquito C, Rampon O, De Rossi A. (2006). Antiretroviral therapy for prevention of mother-to-child transmission: focus on single-dose nevirapine. Clinical Drug investigation, 26(11):611-27.

Graneheim, U.N., Lundman, B., (2004). Qualitative content analysis in nursing research: concepts, procedures and measures to achieve trustworthiness, *Nurse education today, 24, 105 -112.*

Halkin JS *et al.,* (2005). Prevention of mother to child transmission of HIV, Progress and challenges, *Bayloraids organization, curriculum,*

Homsy J, Kalamya JN, Obonyo J, Ojwang J, Mugumya R, Opio C, Mermin J. (2006). Routine intrapartum HIV counseling and testing for prevention of mother -to-child transmission of HIV in a rural Ugandan Hospital, Journal of Acquired Immune Deficiency syndrome, 42(2):149-54.

Hilgert NI, Gil GE. (2007). Reproductive medicine in northwest Argentina: traditional and institutional systems, Journal of Ethnobiology and Ethnomedicine, 3(1):19.

IRIN. (2007). Malawi: Limping PMTCT programme failing infants. UN office of the coordination of humanitarian affairs, IRIN Africa, Southern Africa, Malawi.

Kakimoto K, Kana K, Mukoyama Y, Chheng TV, Chou TL, Sedtha C. (2007). Influence of the involvement of partners in the mother class with voluntary confidential counseling and testing acceptance for prevention of mother to child transmission of HIV programme (PMTCT programme) in Cambodia, AIDS Care, 19(3):381-4.

Kamatenesi-Mugisha M, Oryem-Origa H. (2006). Medicinal plants used to induce labour during childbirth in western Uganda, Journal of Ethnopharmacology, 109(1):1-9.

Loss J, Eichhorn C, Gehlert J, Donhauser J, Wise M, Nagel E. (2007). Community -based health promotion- a change for the evaluation, Gesundheitswesen, 69(2):77-87.

Lallemant M *et al.,* (2004). Single dose perinatal nevirapine plus standard zidovudine to prevent mother to child transmission of HIV-1 in Thailand, *The New England Journal of Medicine, volume 251:217-228 (3)*

Maharaj P, Cleland J. (2005). Women on top: the relative influence of wives and husbands on contraceptive use in Kwazulu-Natal, Women Health, 41 (2):31-41.

Mant J, Winner S, Roche J, Wade DT. (2005). Family support for stroke: one year follow up of a randomized controlled trial, Journal of Neurology, Neurosurgery and Psychiatry, 76(7):1006-8.

Mathole T, Lindmark G, Ahlberg BM. (2005). Competing knowledge claims in the provision of antenatal care: a qualitative study of traditional birth attendants in rural Zimbabwe, Health Care for Women International, 26 (10): 937-56.

MDHS, (2004). Malawi Demographic and Health survey, HIV/AIDS Prevalence, National Statistics Office, *Demography and Social Statistics Division, Zomba.*

Moodley J, Moodley D. (2005). Best practice and research, Clinical obstetrics and gynaecology, 19(2):169-183.

Mshana GH, Wamoyi J, Busza J et. al. (2006). Barriers to accessing antiretroviral therapy in Kisesa, Tanzania: a qualitative study of early rural referrals to the national program. AIDS Patient Care and STDS, 20(9):649-57.

Newell ML. (2006). Current issues in the transmission of mother-to-child transmission of HIV-1 infection. Transactions of Royal Society of Tropical Medicine and Hygiene, 100(1):1-5.

Open Code 3.4 © 2007, UMDAC and Division of Epidemiology and Public Health Sciences, Department of Public Health and Clinical Medicine, Umeå University, Sweden. Website: http://www.umu.se/phmed/epidemi/forskning/open_code.html

Owens, RA. (2006). The caring behaviors of the home health nurses and influence on medication adherence, Home Healthcare Nurse, 24 (8):517-26.

Santelli JS, Speizer IS, Avery A, Kendall C. (2006). An exploration of the dimensions of pregnancy intentions among women choosing to terminate pregnancy or to initiate prenatal care in New Orleans, Louisiana, American Journal of Public Health, 96 (11):2009-15.

Scarlatti G. (2004). Mother -to-child of HIV-1: advances and controversies of the twentieth centuries. AIDS review, AIDS review, 6(2):67-78.

UNAIDS. (2006).Malawi: HIV/AIDS Estimates, Uniting the world against AIDS, Geneva.

6

HIV/AIDS Among Immigrants in Portugal: Socio-Demographic and Behavioural Correlates of Preventive Practices

Sónia Dias, Ana Gama and Maria O. Martins
Instituto de Higiene e Medicina Tropical/Universidade Nova de Lisboa
Portugal

1. Introduction

HIV infection remains a major public health concern in Europe, with evidence of continuing transmission of HIV. Surveillance data published by the European Centre for Disease Prevention and Control and the World Health Organization Regional Office for Europe indicate that, in 2009, 53 427 cases of HIV were diagnosed and reported by 49 of the 53 countries in the WHO European Region; the rate of HIV cases diagnosed was 8.5 per 100 000 population in this region (European Centre for Disease Prevention and Control/World Health Organization Regional Office for Europe [ECDC/WHO Regional Office for Europe], 2010). Migration has been acknowledged as a factor influencing the epidemiology of HIV in Europe (ECDC, 2010a). In 2005, 46% of all cases of heterosexually acquired HIV infection in Western Europe involved migrants from high prevalence countries (ECDC, 2009).

Portugal is one of the western European countries with the highest burden of HIV infection (European Centre for the Epidemiological Monitoring of AIDS [EuroHIV], 2007). Recent data estimates that, in 2007, Portugal presented one of the highest rates of new HIV diagnosis in the European Region (ECDC/WHO Regional Office for Europe, 2008). The epidemic has been mainly driven by injecting drug users, but recently sexually transmitted cases are on the rise.

The Portuguese epidemic is of the concentrated type, i.e. prevalence within the general Portuguese is inferior to 1% but specific groups present a high prevalence of HIV infection (National Coordination for HIV/AIDS Infection, 2007). The groups considered most vulnerable, characterized by a more intensive and frequent exposure and by a more difficult access to means of prevention, include the migrants (National Coordination for HIV/AIDS Infection, 2007). In fact, estimates indicate that immigrants represent approximately 20% of Portugal's diagnosed HIV cases, accounting for a disproportionate number of new heterosexually acquired infections (ECDC, 2010a).

In the last decades, immigrants' inflows have increased across most OECD countries (Organisation for Economic Co-operation and Development [OECD], 2011). Statistics on international migration in the European Union (EU) estimate that, in 2008, the total number of non-nationals (people who are not citizens of their country of residence) living on the territory of the EU Member States was 31.8 million, representing 6.4% of the EU's population (Eurostat, 2010). Around two thirds of all non-nationals living in the EU were citizens of a third country (non-EU Member State).

The proportion of immigrants in Portugal has also continuously increasing. According to recent data, the total stock of foreign population (with a valid residence permit) reached 457 000 in 2009 (4.3% of the total population) (OECD, 2011). Most of these immigrants have come from Brazil, Ukraine and Cape Verde (OECD, 2011).

Migration places populations in situations of greater risk for poor health in general and HIV in particular (ECDC, 2010a; WHO, 2010). The linkages between migration and HIV/Aids are largely related to the conditions and structures of the migration process itself, as in the countries of origin, transit and destination (International Organization for Migration [IOM], 2006). In host countries specifically, factors like poverty, exploitation, lack of legal protection, social exclusion and discrimination may increase the risk of exposure to HIV and may reduce the individual's ability to protect him- or herself from infection (Fenton, 2001; Soskolne & Shtarkshall, 2002). Other potential risk factors for migrants include separation from families and partners, besides separation from the socio-cultural norms that guide behaviours in more stable communities. These circumstances may reinforce the adoption of risk behaviours such as consumption of injection drugs and sexual risk practices (Albarrán & Nyamathi, 2011). Additionally, immigration policies that make integration of migrants in host countries more difficult may have a negative impact on their health (Grove, 2006). In fact, health vulnerability of migrants has been associated to poor access to health care (Derose et al., 2009; Politzer et al., 2001; Stronks et al., 2001). Barriers to health services, including legal, socioeconomic, linguistic and cultural constraints, may result in a reduced utilization of services, in particular for HIV/Aids prevention and care, which makes these groups more vulnerable to HIV and their related complications (Dias et al., 2004; Salama & Dondero, 2001).

Increasing the uptake of HIV testing has been acknowledgedly an important component of primary and secondary prevention strategies (Burns et al., 2005; ECDC, 2010b). Timely HIV testing may lead to improved clinical outcomes through early diagnosis and access to treatment as antiretroviral therapy makes individuals less infectious (Levy et al., 2007; Saracino et al., 2005). Moreover, awareness of positive serostatus may prevent ongoing transmission of disease as it enhances individual behavioural change toward reduced risky sexual behaviour (Ehrlich et al., 2007; Schwarcz et al., 2006).

Given the epidemiological situation in Portugal, national HIV prevention and control efforts targeted to groups most-at-risk as the migrant population have been a priority. During the last decade, one of the main strategies undertaken has been generalizing access to early detection of the infection and promotion of voluntary testing and counselling (National Coordination for HIV/AIDS Infection, 2007). Presently, HIV testing in Portugal is non-mandatory and can be done anonymously, confidentially and for free at the HIV Early Detection and Counselling Centres.

Despite the benefits of HIV testing upon the individual and the community, and the continued efforts to guarantee access to diagnosis and promote the uptake of HIV testing in Portugal, a high proportion of adults in this country remain so far untested (National Coordination for HIV/AIDS Infection, 2007). Since 2001, immigrants in Portugal are entitled to health care regardless of legal status, including free health care to pregnant women and recent mothers, users of family planning programmes and individuals with transmissible diseases. Nevertheless, evidence on access and utilization of health services among migrants in Portugal suggests that barriers related to legal issues, economic constraints, lack of information of migrants on their health rights and negative attitudes of health professionals remain (Dias et al., 2008, 2010a).

Knowledge on HIV testing among immigrants is limited; nevertheless, the literature indicates that a proportion of these groups remain undiagnosed and tend to utilize HIV health services at a later stage of disease (Burns et al., 2007; Delpierre et al., 2007). A growing body of literature indicates that factors such as socio-demographic (sex, age, country of origin, education, immigration status), behavioural (perceived risk for HIV, risk behaviours) and structural (utilization of health services) are associated with HIV testing (Bond et al., 2005; Stein & Nyamathi, 2000; Stolte et al., 2003; Wang et al., 2010).

Understanding such factors among immigrants may contribute to developing strategies designed to effectively promote HIV testing and reduce undiagnosed infection. This paper aims to describe the proportion of HIV testing among an immigrant population in Portugal and identify demographic, socioeconomic, behavioural and structural factors.

2. Methods

Based on a participatory approach, a cross-sectional study was conducted with a sample of 1282 immigrants (35.7% from Portuguese-speaking African countries, 33.2% from Eastern European countries and 31.1% from Brazil) living in the Lisbon Metropolitan Area. This area has currently the highest concentration of immigrant population in the country. Official data indicate that, in 2010, 43% of the immigrant population in Portugal (around 189 220 immigrants) resided in the Lisbon region (Serviço de Estrangeiros e Fronteiras, 2011).

2.1 Sampling and data collection

Participants were selected through snowball sampling. This sampling method was used as the information available on immigrant population in Portugal does not allow constructing sampling frames for representative population based surveys.

Representatives of non-governmental organisations (NGOs) and associations of African, Brazilian and eastern European immigrants were contacted by the research team and invited to collaborate in the study. The investigators carried out several meetings with NGOs members to present the research' main objectives and procedures and ask their collaboration in publicising the study within the immigrant community and in identifying and recruiting potential participants. The inclusion criteria were being an immigrant, defined as a non-national person who migrated for settlement purposes (IOM, 2004) and being 18 years old or older. These potential participants were personally approached and invited to participate by the research team. After respondents finished filling the questionnaire they were asked to identify and recruit within their social networks other possible participants who met the study criteria.

Data was collected between May 2010 and January 2011 through a questionnaire applied in community based associations, governmental and non-governmental organizations working with immigrant populations. Data collection days were scheduled with these entities based on the availability of free rooms for that purpose. Given the sensitive nature of the subject under investigation, the questionnaires were administered in a quiet room, in isolation, to ensure privacy and comfort of participants.

Questionnaires were applied by trained interviewers from immigrant communities, recruited and selected in collaboration with NGOs and immigrant associations. The interviewers training included information about the questionnaire, the data collection procedures and general interview techniques. A training manual was elaborated and provided to support interviewers in the field.

The questionnaire comprised closed-ended questions on sociodemographics, self-perception of HIV risk, knowing someone infected, number of sexual partners in Portugal in the last 12 months, having had a consultation on sexual and reproductive health, and HIV testing. The instrument of data collection was constructed along with feedback provided by partners of the study - community based associations, governmental and non-governmental organizations. After the questionnaire was developed, a pre-test was conducted with members of immigrant communities; few amendments were made to improve clarity of the questions and to make it better adapted to the study populations.

Anonymous participation and confidentiality of data was guaranteed. Informed consent was obtained. The study was approved by the Ethical Committee of the Institute of Hygiene and Tropical Medicine, New University of Lisbon.

2.2 Measures

Sociodemographic characteristics included sex, age (continuous variable), origin ('African', 'Brazilian', 'Eastern European'), educational level ('elementary education', 'secondary education', 'higher education'), immigration status ('legal status', 'irregular status'). Length of stay was a continuous variable measured in years.

Self-perception of HIV risk was measured using a dichotomous question on fearing to become infected with HIV ('yes'/'no'). Knowing someone infected (friend or relative) had also two response options: 'yes'/'no'. The number of sexual partners in Portugal in the last 12 months was a continuous variable; for descriptive analysis, this variable was recoded into a three-category variable: '1 sexual partner', '2-4 sexual partners' and '≥ 5 sexual partners'.

Having had a consultation on sexual and reproductive health, having ever been tested for HIV, having been tested in Portugal and having been tested in the last year were measured as dichotomous variables ('yes'/'no').

2.3 Data analysis

Descriptive analysis was conducted for background characteristics of participants; continuous variables are presented as mean ± standard deviation. The associations between socio-demographic characteristics, fear of becoming infected, knowing someone infected, number of sexual partners, having had a consultation on sexual and reproductive health, HIV testing and the three immigrant groups were analysed using the Chi-Square test (for categorical variables) and the Kruskal-Wallis test (for continuous variables).

A logistic regression analysis was performed to identify factors associated with having ever been HIV tested. In the final model, all the variables that were found to be significantly associated with HIV testing were included: age, sex, origin, educational level, fear of becoming infected, knowing someone infected, number of sexual partners and having had a consultation on sexual and reproductive health. The magnitude of the associations was estimated by means of odds ratios (OR) with 95% confidence intervals. The software SPSS 18.0 was used for all the data analysis.

3. Results

3.1 Socio-demographic characteristics of participants

Of the total sample, more than a half was female (Table 1). Eastern Europeans were significantly older than Africans and Brazilians. Differences on educational level were found across origin. Most participants reported to have legal status, more frequently Eastern Europeans than Brazilians and Africans. The mean length of stay was higher among Africans, compared to Eastern Europeans and Brazilians (Table 1).

	Total		African		Brazilian		Eastern European		*P value*
	n	%	n	%	n	%	n	%	
Sex									
Female	715	55.8	265	57.9	235	55.2	215	54.0	0.504
Male	567	44.2	193	42.1	191	44.8	183	46.0	
Educational level									
Elementary education	356	27.9	269	58.7	61	14.3	26	6.6	
Secondary education	480	37.6	116	25.3	258	60.6	106	27.0	<0.001
Higher education	441	34.5	73	15.9	107	25.1	261	66.4	
Immigration status									
Legal	1088	86.0	372	82.5	356	84.4	360	91.8	<0.001
Irregular	177	14.0	79	17.5	66	15.6	32	8.2	
	Mean	SD	Mean	SD	Mean	SD	Mean	SD	
Age (years)	35.4	10.6	35.5	11.0	33.8	9.8	37.1	10.8	<0.001
Length of stay (years)	7.9	10.2	11.6	10.2	4.1	6.1	7.8	11.9	<0.001

Table 1. Socio-demographic characteristics of participants

3.2 HIV risk perception, knowing someone infected and number of sexual partners

Most participants (59.6%) referred to fear becoming infected with HIV, more frequently Brazilians (69.7%) and Africans (65.8%) compared to Eastern Europeans (41.6%) ($p<0.001$) (Table 2). Differences were found across sex: a higher proportion of women feared becoming infected compared to men (63.2% vs. 55.0%, respectively) ($p=0.003$). Origin differences across sexes remained: Brazilian and African women reported more often to fear becoming infected compared to Eastern European women (73.1% and 68.1% vs. 46.2%) ($p<0.001$), as Brazilian and African men reported more often fearing to become infected than Eastern European men (65.6% and 62.6% vs. 36.1%) ($p<0.001$).

Almost 28% of participants had a friend or relative infected with HIV, more frequently Brazilians (35.7%) and Africans (25.9%) than Eastern Europeans (19.1%) ($p<0.001$) (Table 2). Knowing someone infected did not differ significantly between men and women.

The mean number of sexual partners in Portugal in the last 12 months was 1.6 ± 4.2; 70% of participants referred having had one sexual partner, 19% had between two and four and 11% had five or more sexual partners (Table 2). Brazilians reported more frequently to have had one sexual partner in the last 12 months (73.4% vs. 68.7% Africans and 67.4% Eastern Europeans); Africans reported more frequently having had between two and four partners (22.2% vs. 20.1% Brazilians and 14.5% Eastern Europeans); Eastern Europeans reported more frequently to having had five or more sexual partners (18.1% vs. 9.1% Africans and 6.5% Brazilians) ($p<0.001$) (Table 2). Differences by sex were also found, with women reporting more often to have one sexual partner than men (80.6% vs. 57.9%) and men reporting more frequently higher number of sexual partners than women (2-4 partners: 28.7% vs. 10.6%; ≥ 5 partners: 13.4% vs. 8.9%) ($p<0.001$). In each sex group, the number of sexual partners in Portugal in the last year differed across origins. Among women, more frequently Africans and Brazilians referred having one sexual partner (84.9% and 83.3%, respectively, vs. 71.9% Eastern Europeans), Brazilians having between two and four (13.1% vs. 9.8% Eastern Europeans and 8.4% Africans) and Eastern Europeans having more than four partners (18.3% vs. 6.7% Africans and 3.5% Brazilians) ($p<0.001$). In contrast, among men, more frequently Eastern Europeans and Brazilians reported having one sexual partner (63.1% and 60.9%, respectively, vs. 49.3% Africans), Africans having between two and four (38.7% vs. 28.8% Brazilians and 19.1% Eastern Europeans) and Eastern Europeans having more than four (17.8% vs. 12% Africans and 10.3% Brazilians) ($p=0.002$).

	Total		African		Brazilian		Eastern European		*P value*
	n	%	n	%	n	%	n	%	
Fear of becoming infected with HIV									
Yes	752	59.6	294	65.8	295	69.7	163	41.6	<0.001
No	510	40.4	153	34.2	128	30.3	229	58.4	
Knowing someone infected with HIV									
Yes	322	27.5	113	25.9	148	35.7	61	19.1	<0.001
No	850	72.5	324	74.1	267	64.3	259	80.9	
	Mean	SD	Mean	SD	Mean	SD	Mean	SD	
Number of sexual partners in Portugal in the last 12 months	1.6	4.2	1.9	6.0	1.5	2.4	1.2	2.8	0.094

Table 2. HIV risk perception, knowing someone infected and number of sexual partners

3.3 Consultation on sexual and reproductive health and HIV testing

Of the total sample, having been tested for HIV at least once was reported by 60%; more frequently among Brazilians (73.2%) and Africans (63.5%) than Eastern Europeans (41.9%) ($p<0.001$) (Table 3). Across sex, a significantly higher proportion of women had been HIV tested compared to men (63.4% vs. 55.8%) ($p=0.006$). Differences on having ever been tested for HIV across origins remained among women and men (women: 72.6% Brazilians and 70.2% Africans vs. 44.9% Eastern Europeans; $p<0.001$) (men: 73.8% Brazilians and 54.4% Africans vs. 38.5% Eastern Europeans; $p<0.001$). No differences were observed across immigration status.

Having ever been HIV tested was mainly due to routine medical screening (31.2%), pregnancy/partners' pregnancy (20.2%), curiosity (12.6%), requirement for mortgage or life/health insurance application (6.4%) and having engaged in risk behaviours (6%). Of those participants who were never tested, the main reasons were having never had risk behaviours (28.6%), not thinking about it (19.6%), not perceiving to be at risk (16.3%), feeling well (11.7%), not knowing where to do the test (9.3%) and not considering it important (6.9%).

Among those who have ever been tested for HIV, 54.6% had a test in Portugal; 77.4% of Africans versus 42.3% Eastern Europeans and 39.7% Brazilians ($p<0.001$) (Table 3). Having been tested in Portugal did not differ significantly between women and men.

Of participants who have ever been tested, 36.8% had their last test in the previous year (Table 3). Having been tested in the last year was more frequent among Africans (41.2% vs. 36.5% Brazilians and 29.7% Eastern Europeans) ($p=0.048$). Also, HIV testing was more frequent among women (39.7% vs. 32.7%) ($p=0.048$). In both sex groups, origin differences were not found regarding having been tested in the last year.

Approximately 23% of participants referred having had a consultation on sexual and reproductive health; no differences were found across origin (Table 3). According to sex, a higher proportion of women had a sexual and reproductive health consultation compared to men (32% vs. 12.4%) ($p<0.001$).

	Total		African		Brazilian		Eastern European		*P value*
	n	%	n	%	n	%	n	%	
Having ever been tested for HIV									
Yes	768	60.0	291	63.5	311	73.2	166	41.9	<0.001
No	511	40.0	167	36.5	114	26.8	230	58.1	
Having been tested in Portugal									
Yes	412	54.6	223	77.4	123	39.7	66	42.3	<0.001
No	342	45.4	65	22.6	187	60.3	90	57.7	
Having been tested in the last year									
Yes	282	36.8	120	41.2	113	36.5	49	29.7	0.048
No	484	63.2	171	58.8	197	63.5	116	70.3	
Having ever had a consultation on sexual and reproductive health									
Yes	295	23.3	105	23.1	90	21.2	100	25.9	0.288
No	969	76.7	349	76.9	334	78.8	286	74.1	

Table 3. HIV testing (ever, in Portugal and in the last year) and consultation on sexual and reproductive health

3.4 Factors associated with HIV testing

The logistic regression analysis allowed the identification of sex, origin, fear of becoming infected with HIV, knowing someone infected, number of sexual partners and having ever had a consultation on sexual and reproductive health as positively associated with having been tested for HIV.

After adjusting for potential confounding factors, having ever been tested was positively associated with being older (OR = 1.02, CI 95% = [1.01-1.03]), female (OR = 1.39, CI 95% = [1.05-1.84]), Brazilian (OR = 3.75, CI 95% = [2.56-5.50]) and African (OR = 2.60, CI 95% = [1.75-3.86]) compared to Eastern European, and having higher education (OR = 1.55, CI 95% = [1.04-2.31]) compared to elementary education (Table 4). HIV testing was also more likely among those reporting fear to become infected with HIV (OR = 1.28, CI 95% = [0.97-1.70]; $p<0.10$), knowing someone infected (OR = 1.97, CI 95% = [1.43-2.71]), having higher number

	Crude OR (CI 95%)	*P value*	Adjusted OR (CI 95%)	*P value*
Age	1.00 (0.99-1.01)	0.806	1.02 (1.01-1.03)	0.005*
Sex				
Male	1		1	
Female	1.37 (1.09-1.72)	0.006*	1.39 (1.05-1.84)	0.022*
Origin				
Eastern European	1		1	
African	2.41 (1.83-3.18)	<0.001*	2.60 (1.75-3.86)	<0.001*
Brazilian	3.78 (2.82-5.07)	<0.001*	3.75 (2.56-5.50)	<0.001*
Educational level				
Elementary education	1		1	
Secondary education	0.98 (0.74-1.30)	0.903	1.06 (0.74-1.52)	0.763
Higher education	0.80 (0.60-1.06)	0.120	1.55 (1.04-2.31)	0.033*
Immigration status				
Non regular	1		1	
Regular	0.97 (0.70-1.35)	0.870	1.29 (0.89-1.87)	0.183
Fear of becoming infected with HIV				
No	1		1	
Yes	1.96 (1.56-2.47)	<0.001*	1.28 (0.97-1.70)	0.084**
Knowing someone infected with HIV				
No	1		1	
Yes	2.35 (1.76-3.13)	<0.001*	1.97 (1.43-2.71)	<0.001*
Number of sexual partners	1.15 (1.06-1.25)	0.001*	1.12 (1.03-1.22)	0.008*
Having ever had a consultation on sexual and reproductive health				
No	1		1	
Yes	2.37 (1.77-3.18)	<0.001*	2.52 (1.78-3.58)	<0.001*

*Statistically significant at $p<0.05$
**Statistically significant at $p<0.10$

Table 4. Factors associated with HIV testing

of sexual partners (OR = 1.12, CI 95% = [1.03-1.22]) and having ever had a consultation on sexual and reproductive health (OR = 2.52, CI 95% = [1.78-3.58]). No significant association was found between HIV testing and immigration status.

4. Conclusion

In this study, the prevalence of having ever been tested for HIV was 58.6%, higher than the one (51.2%) estimated in a previous study conducted in 2007 with a sample of immigrants residing in Lisbon (Dias et al., 2010b). The prevalence of HIV testing obtained in the present study was also higher compared to the one estimated in the National Survey of Sexual Behaviour conducted in 2009 - 44% of a representative sample of the general Portuguese population aged 16-64 years old reported having been tested for HIV (National Coordination for HIV/AIDS Infection). The findings of the present study may indicate that the national efforts undertaken during the last years to promote HIV testing among most-at-risk groups as migrants have been positive.

The most commonly reported motivations for having been tested were event-driven (routine medical screening, pregnancy or partners' pregnancy). Also, approximately a fifth of participants were tested based on person-driven reasons (i.e., having the desire to know one's own HIV serostatus, having engaged in risk behaviours). This result may reflect the positive outcomes of prevention strategies population-wide focused on increasing awareness of the importance of doing the test. Nevertheless, reported reasons for having never been tested included low self-risk perception and lack of information on where HIV test can be done. These findings reinforce that continuing efforts are needed to encourage HIV testing among immigrant population.

In this study, demographic, socioeconomic, behavioural and structural factors were identified as predictors of HIV testing.

Differences observed across sex are consistent with previous research reporting higher prevalence of HIV testing among women (Fakoya et al., 2008; Lopez-Quintero et al., 2005). This may be due to the fact that migrant women are commonly of reproductive age and therefore tend to use more health services than men (Bond et al., 2005; Dias et al., 2008). Indeed, in this study, having had a consultation on sexual and reproductive health was more often reported by women. Currently, universal prenatal care in Portugal includes HIV counselling and testing. This may result in more opportunities to get information on HIV prevention and to uptake the test among female migrants.

Accordingly, having had a sexual and reproductive health consultation was also positively associated with HIV testing. Although reasons for having never been consulted were not explored, the results suggest that access to health services is important in linking individuals with HIV testing services. In previous studies, utilization of health services has been found to increase the likelihood of HIV detection as these services are a useful setting in which to provide HIV preventive counselling and promote HIV testing (Bond et al., 2005; Wang et al., 2010). The findings may also suggest that health professionals may be influential in encouraging individuals to receive HIV testing. In fact, previous studies have shown that HIV testing is more likely when health care providers initiate discussion, emphasize its benefits and strongly recommend it (Fernandez et al., 2000).

Age and educational level were also significant socioeconomic factors of HIV testing, similarly to other studies (Fernández et al., 2005; Haile et al., 2007). Higher education has been positively associated with HIV knowledge, awareness of availability of health services and HIV testing (Burns et al., 2005; Dias et al., 2004; Stolte et al., 2003; Wong et al., 2004).

The results show a significant variation across origins, with Brazilian and African participants reporting more often to have been tested for HIV. A similar result was obtained in a previous study (Dias et al., 2010b). In the countries of origin of these participants, Portuguese is the official language. This may reinforce the idea that having a common language may be a facilitator of utilization of health services, and in particular for HIV testing. In several other investigations, linguistic differences have been mentioned as predictive of underutilization of HIV-related health services and having never been tested for HIV among immigrants (Burns et al., 2007; Dias et al., 2004; Prost et al., 2008).

In this study, having been tested for HIV appeared to be independent of immigration status, which may reflect the efforts undertaken to promote voluntary, anonymous and confidential HIV testing, free of charge and regardless of legal status (National Coordination for HIV/AIDS Infection, 2007).

Two thirds of participants feared becoming HIV infected; this variable was associated with higher odds of having been tested for HIV. Perception of individual HIV risk has been associated with knowledge of HIV risk factors, fewer risk-taking practices and HIV testing (Bardem-O'Fallon et al., 2004; Maman et al., 2001; Stein & Nyamathi, 2000). It is possible that individuals who perceive to be at risk for HIV infection are more likely to consider the disease as a personal danger, to recognize its consequences and to acknowledge the importance of adopting HIV-related protective measures (Norman & Gebre, 2005; Worthington & Myers, 2003). Differences by origin revealed that Brazilians and Africans report a higher perception of HIV risk, compared to Eastern Europeans. These findings are consistent with research suggesting that migrants from high prevalence countries tend to show high levels of knowledge and awareness of HIV risk factors (Burns et al., 2007). These migrants may therefore be more likely to perceive themselves at risk of HIV infection. Women also reported higher perception of individual risk compared to men. Although reasons for fearing to become infected with HIV were not explored in this study, in previous investigations the lack of trust in a male partner and a partner's promiscuity are the most common reasons given for perceived high personal risk (Dias et al., 2004, 2010c; Sarker et al., 2005; Ventura-Filipe et al., 2000). Additional research is needed to deepen understanding of the ways in which issues of gender and origin underpin HIV risk perception.

The results show a significant association between knowing someone infected and HIV testing. Studies have pointed out that knowing someone with HIV/AIDS appears to be an important contributor to knowledge of HIV and may result in more positive attitudes toward HIV protective measures (Barden-O'Fallon et al., 2004; Kalichman & Simbayi, 2003). Increased knowledge and more positive attitudes may help individuals to recognize the benefits of the HIV test (Norman & Gebre, 2005). The differences observed by origin support the hypothesis that country of origin's background plays an important role in HIV-related perceptions and experiences, thus influencing willingness to test for HIV.

In this study, risky sexual behaviour as having multiple sexual partners was a predictor of HIV testing. This result confirms the findings of surveys conducted in other countries showing that increasing number of sexual partners is associated with progressively higher prevalence of testing (Song et al., 2011; Wang et al., 2010). When individuals experience sexual risk behaviours, they may be aware of their increased risk for HIV infection and, in turn, they may be more likely to test for HIV. The findings indicate a variation on sexual behaviour patterns across origin and sex. Further investigation on sexual behaviours must take into account the cultural and gender-related influences.

This study points out interesting challenges for HIV prevention among immigrants and may help in the design of tailored interventions focused on promotion of HIV testing among these populations. The findings highlight that strategies should be targeted to specific subgroups including men, Eastern Europeans, those younger, with lower educational level and in stable relationships.

In view of the missed opportunities for HIV testing in outpatient care, this study reinforces that the sexual and reproductive health services may be a useful setting in which to provide HIV preventive counselling and testing. These services are considered to greatly contribute to HIV prevention given their potential outreach to diverse groups of the population through primary health care (Berer, 2004). Voluntary counselling in primary care is increasingly recognized as an appropriate way to encourage early diagnosis of HIV among immigrants, many of whom often do not suspect to be infected (Askew & Berer, 2003). Interventions might therefore focus on improving the provision of HIV information, counselling and testing in primary care.

Further efforts to improve HIV testing among immigrants should focus on increasing individuals' awareness of HIV self-risk and benefits of doing the test, as well as on promoting utilization of health services and providing access to timely, culturally competent and appropriate HIV testing and counselling.

Studies have consistently pointed toward the need for creating further innovative and effective pathways to HIV testing of immigrant populations (Burns et al., 2001; Delpierre et al., 2007; Erwin et al., 2002). The provision of HIV detection services in non-traditional health settings such as mobile units may be important to facilitate HIV testing and dissemination of HIV information within immigrant communities. Also, the role of community based organizations in HIV prevention among 'hard-to-reach' populations as immigrants has been increasingly recognized (Fakoya et al., 2008; Solorio et al., 2004). Community-based organizations may provide counselling and testing services to migrants and may link those testing positive with health care services, increasing timely access to treatment and care. These organizations may also provide culturally relevant information on HIV risks, protective measures and health services available. Communities' involvement and participation in the planning and development of HIV prevention interventions should be supported.

A deeper understanding of the individual, behavioural and structural factors that underpin HIV testing among immigrant populations is needed. Cultural and gender-related issues should be taken into account as contributors for variation in sexual behaviour patterns, adoption of protective measures and HIV testing across immigrant groups. This knowledge is relevant to support the design of interventions aimed to increase access to diagnosis and reduce the proportion of undiagnosed HIV infection.

5. Acknowledgment

This work was partially supported by National Coordination for HIV/AIDS Infection. The authors wish to thank all participants of this study. The authors also would like to acknowledge the commitment of the team of interviewers who were responsible for the collection of the study data.

6. References

Albarrán, C.R., & Nyamathi, A. (2011). HIV and Mexican Migrant Workers in the United States: A Review Applying the Vulnerable Populations Conceptual Model. *Journal of the Association of Nurses in AIDS Care*, Vol.22, No.3, (May-June 2011), pp. 173-185, ISSN 1055-3290

Askew, I., & Berer, M. (2003). The Contribution of Sexual and Reproductive Health Services to the Fight Against HIV/AIDS: A Review. *Reproductive Health Matters*, Vol.11, No.22, (November 2003), pp. 51-73, ISSN 1460-9576

Barden-O'Fallon, J.L., deGraft-Johnson, J., Bisika, T., Sulzbach, S., Benson, A., & Tsui, A.O. (2004). Factors Associated with HIV/AIDS Knowledge and Risk Perception in Rural Malawi. *AIDS and Behavior*, Vol.8, No.2, (June 2004), pp. 131-140, ISSN 1573-3254

Berer, M. (2004). HIV/AIDS, Sexual and Reproductive Health: Intersections and Implications for National Programmes. *Health Policy and Planning*, Vol.19, Suppl.1, (October 2004), pp. i62–i70, ISSN 1460-2237

Bond, L., Lauby, J., & Batson, H. (2005). HIV Testing and the Role of Individual- and Structural-level Barriers and Facilitators. *AIDS Care*, Vol.17, No.2, (February 2005), pp. 125-140, ISSN 1360-0451

Burns, F., Imrie, J., Nazroo, J., Johnson, A., & Fenton, K. (2007). Why The(y) Wait? Key Informant Understandings of Factors Contributing to Late Presentation and Poor Utilization of HIV Health and Social Care Services by African Migrants in Britain. *AIDS Care*, Vol.19, No.1, (January 2007), pp. 102-108, ISSN 1360-0451

Burns, F., Fenton, K.A., Morison, L., Mercer, C., Erens, B., Field, J., Copas, A.J., Wellings, K., & Johnson, A. (2005). Factors Associated with HIV Testing Among Black Africans in Britain. *Sexually Transmitted Infections*, Vol.81, No.6, (December 2005), pp. 494-500, ISSN 1368-4973

Burns, F.M., Fakoya, A.O., Copas, A.J., & French, P.D. (2001). Africans in London Continue to Present with Advanced HIV Disease in the Era of Highly Active Antiretroviral Therapy. *AIDS*, Vol.15, No.18, (December 2001), pp. 2453-2455, ISSN 0269-9370

Delpierre, C., Dray-Spira, R., Cuzin, L., Marchou, B., Massip, P., Lang, T., Lert, F., & The Vespa Study Group (2007). Correlates of Late HIV Diagnosis: Implications for Testing Policy. *International Journal of STD and AIDS*, Vol.18, No.5, (May 2007), pp. 312-317, ISSN 1758-1052

Derose, K.P., Bahney, B.W., Lurie, N., & Escarce, J.J. (2009). Immigrants and Health Care Access, Quality, and Cost. *Medical Care Research and Review*, Vol.66, No.4, (August 2009), pp. 355-408. ISSN 1552-6801

Dias, S., Gonçalves, A., Luck, M., & Fernandes, M. (2004). [Risk of HIV/AIDS Infection: Access and Utilization of Health Services in a Migrant Community]. *Acta Médica Portuguesa*, Vol.17, No.3, (May-June 2004), pp. 211-218, ISSN 0870-399x

Dias, S., Severo, M., & Barros, H. (2008). Determinants of Health Care Utilization by Immigrants in Portugal. *BMC Health Services Research*, Vol.8, (October 2008), pp. 207, [Epub ahead of print], ISSN 1472-6963

Dias, S., Gama, A., & Rocha, C. (2010a). Immigrant Women's Perceptions and Experiences of Health Care Services: Insights from a Focus Group Study. *Journal of Public Health*, Vol.18, No.5, (October 2010), pp. 489-496, ISSN 1613-2238

Dias, S., Gama, A., Severo, M., & Barros, H. (2010b). Factors Associated with HIV Testing Among Immigrants in Portugal. *International Journal of Public Health*, (November 2010), [Epub ahead of print], ISSN 1661-8564

Dias, S., Gama, A., & Rocha, C. (2010c). Perspectives of African and Brazilian Immigrant Women on Sexual and Reproductive Health. *European Journal of Contraception and Reproductive Health Care*, Vol.15, No.4, (August 2010), pp. 255–263, ISSN 1473-0782

ECDC (July 2009). *Migrant Health Series: Background Note to the 'ECDC Report on Migration and Infectious Diseases in the EU'*, 23.03.2011, Available from http://ecdc.europa.eu/en/publications/Publications/0907_TER_Migrant_health_Background_note.pdf

ECDC (2010a). *Migrant Health Series: Epidemiology of HIV and AIDS in Migrant Communities and Ethnic Minorities in EU/ EEA countries*, ECDC, ISBN 978-92-9193-204-7, Stockholm, Sweden

ECDC (2010b). *HIV Testing: Increasing Uptake and Effectiveness in the European Union*, ECDC, ISBN 978-92-9193-224-5, Stockholm, Sweden

ECDC/WHO Regional Office for Europe (2008). *HIV/AIDS Surveillance in Europe 2007*, ECDC, ISBN 978-92-9193-139-2, Stockholm, Sweden

ECDC/WHO Regional Office for Europe (2010). *HIV/AIDS Surveillance in Europe 2009*, ECDC, ISBN 978-92-9193-228-3, Stockholm, Sweden

Ehrlich, S., Organista, K., & Oman, D. (2007). Migrant Latino Day Laborers and Intentions to Test for HIV. *AIDS and Behavior*, Vol.11, No.5, (September 2007), pp. 743-752, ISSN 1573-3254

Erwin, J., Morgan, M., Britten, N., Gray, K., & Peters, B. (2002). Pathways to HIV Testing and Care by Black African and White Patients in London. *Sexually Transmitted Infections*, Vol.78, No.1, (February 2002), pp. 37-39, ISSN 1368-4973

EuroHIV (2007). *HIV/AIDS Surveillance in Europe: End-year Report 2006, No.75*, Institut de Veille Sanitaire, ISSN 1025-8965, Saint-Maurice, France

Eurostat (October 2010). *Migration and Migrant Population Statistics - Statistics Explained*, 26.03.2011, Available from http://epp.eurostat.ec.europa.eu/statistics_explained/
index.php/Migration_and_migrant_population_statistics#

Fakoya, I., Reynolds, R., Caswell, G., & Shiripinda, I. (2008). Barriers to HIV Testing for Migrant Black Africans in Western Europe. *HIV Medicine*, Vol.9, Suppl.2, (July 2008), pp. 23–25, ISSN 1468-1293

Fenton, K. (2001). Strategies for Improving Sexual Health in Ethnic Minorities. *Current Opinion in Infectious Diseases*, Vol.14, No.1, (February 2001), pp. 63-69, ISSN 1535-3877

Fernández, M., Collazo, J., Bowen, S., Varga, L., Hernandez, N., & Perrino, T. (2005). Predictors of HIV Testing and Intention to Test among Hispanic Farmworkers in South Florida. *Journal of Rural Health*, Vol.21, No.1, (Winter 2005), pp. 56-64, ISSN 1748-0361

Fernandez, M.I., Wilson, T.E., Ethier, K.A., Walter, E.B., Gay, C.L., & Moore, J. (2000). Acceptance of HIV Testing During Prenatal Care. Perinatal Guidelines Evaluation Project. *Public Health Reports*, Vol.115, No.5, (September-October 2000), pp. 460-468, ISSN 1468-2877

Grove, N. (2006). Our Health and Theirs: Forced Migration, Othering, and Public Health. *Social Science & Medicine*, Vol.62, No.8, (April 2006), pp. 1931-1942, ISSN 1873-5347

Haile, B., Chambers, J., & Garrison, J. (2007). Correlates of HIV Knowledge and Testing: Results of a 2003 South African Survey. *Journal of Black Studies*, Vol.38, No.2, (November 2007), pp. 194–208, ISSN 0021-9347

IOM (2004). *International Migration Law: Glossary on Migration*, IOM, ISSN 1813-2278, Geneva, Switzerland

IOM (2006). *HIV/AIDS and Populations Mobility: Overview of the IOM Global HIV/AIDS Programme 2006*, 25.04.2011, Available from http://www.iom.int/jahia/webdav/site/myjahiasite/shared/shared/mainsite/published_docs/books/IOM_Global_HIV_pdf.pdf

Kalichman, S., & Simbayi, L. (2003). HIV Testing Attitudes, AIDS Stigma, and Voluntary HIV Counseling and Testing in a Black Township in Cape Town, South Africa. *Sexually Transmitted Infections*, Vol. 79, No. 6, (December 2003), pp. 442-447, ISSN 1368-4973

Levy, V., Prentiss, D., Balmas, G., Chen, S., Israelski, D., Katzenstein, D., & Page-Shafer, K. (2007). Factors in the Delayed HIV Presentation of Immigrants in Northern California: Implications for Voluntary Counselling and Testing Programs. *Journal of Immigrant and Minority Health*, Vol. 9, No.1, (January 2007), pp. 49-54, ISSN 1557-1920

Lopez-Quintero, C., Shtarkshall, R., & Neumark, Y. (2005). Barriers to HIV-testing among Hispanics in the United States: Analysis of the National Health Interview Survey, 2000. *AIDS Patient Care and STDs*, Vol.19, No.10, (October 2005), pp. 672-683, ISSN 1557-7449

Maman, S., Mbwambo, J., Hogan, N.M., Kilonzo, G.P., & Sweat, M. (2001). Women's Barriers to HIV-1 Testing and Disclosure: Challenges for HIV-1 Voluntary Counselling and Testing. *AIDS Care*, Vol.13, No.5, (October 2001), pp. 595–603, ISSN 1360-0451

National Coordination for HIV/AIDS Infection (2007). *National Programme for the Prevention and Control of HIV/AIDS 2007–2010: A Commitment to the Future*, National Coordination for HIV/AIDS Infection, ISBN 978-972-8478-18-6, Lisbon, Portugal

Norman, L., & Gebre, Y. (2005). Prevalence and Correlates of HIV Testing: An Analysis of University Students in Jamaica. *Medscape General Medicine*, Vol.7, No.1, (March 2005), pp. 70, ISSN 1531-0132

OECD (2011). *International Migration Outlook: SOPEMI 2011*, OECD, ISBN 978-92-64-11260-5, Paris, France

Politzer, R.M., Yoon, J., Shi, L., Hughes, R.G., Regan, J., & Gaston, M.H. (2001). Inequality in America: The Contribution of Health Centers in Reducing and Eliminating Disparities in Access to Care. *Medical Care Research Review*, Vol.58, No.2, (June 2001), pp. 234-248, ISSN 1552-6801

Prost, A., Elford, J., Imrie, J., Petticrew, M., & Hart, G.J. (2008). Social, Behavioural, and Intervention Research among People of Sub-Saharan African Origin Living with

HIV in the UK and Europe: Literature Review and Recommendations for Intervention. *AIDS and Behavior*, Vol.12, No.2, (March 2008), pp. 170–194, ISSN 1573-3254

Salama, P., & Dondero, T.J. (2001). HIV Surveillance in Complex Emergencies. *AIDS*, Vol.15, Suppl.3, (April 2001), pp. S4-S12, ISSN 1473-5571

Saracino, A., El-Hamad, I., Prato, R., Cibelli, D., Tartaglia, A., Palumbo, E., Pezzoli, M.C., Angarano, G., Scotto, G., & SIMIT Study Group (2005). Access to HAART in HIV-infected Immigrants: A Retrospective Multicenter Italian Study. *AIDS Patient Care and STDs*, Vol.19, No.9, (September 2005), pp. 599–606, ISSN 1557-7449

Sarker, M., Milkowski, A., Slanger, T., Gondos, A., Sanou, A., Kouyate, B., & Snow, R. (2005). The Role of HIV-Related Knowledge and Ethnicity in Determining HIV Risk Perception and Willingness to Undergo HIV Testing Among Rural Women in Burkina Faso. *AIDS and Behavior*, Vol.9, No.2, (June 2005), pp. 243-249, ISSN 1573-3254

Schwarcz, S., Hsu, L., Dilley, J., Loeb, L., Nelson, K., & Boyd, S. (2006). Late Diagnosis of HIV Infection: Trends, Prevalence, and Characteristics of Persons whose HIV Diagnosis Occurred within 12 Months of Developing AIDS. *Journal of Acquired Immune Deficiency Syndromes*, Vol.43, No.4, (December 2006), pp. 491-494, ISSN 1944-7884

Serviço de Estrangeiros e Fronteiras (2011). *Relatório de Imigração, Fronteiras e Asilo - 2010*, SEF/Departamento de Planeamento e Formação, Lisboa, Portugal

Solorio, M.R., Currier, J., & Cunningham, W. (2004). HIV Health Care Services for Mexican Migrants. *Journal of Acquired Immune Deficiency Syndromes*, Vol.37, Suppl.4, (November 2004), pp. S240–S251, ISSN 1944-7884

Song, Y., Li, X., Zhang, L., Fang, X., Lin, X., Liu, Y., & Stanton, B. (2011). HIV Testing Behavior among Young Migrant Men Who Have Sex With Men (MSM) in Beijing, China. *AIDS Care*, Vol.23, No.2, (February 2011), pp. 179-186, ISSN 1360-0451

Soskolne, V., & Shtarkshall, R.A. (2002). Migration and HIV Prevention Programmes: Linking Structural Factors, Culture, and Individual Behaviour—An Israeli Experience. *Social Science & Medicine*, Vol.55, No.8, (October 2002), pp. 1297-1307, ISSN 1873-5347

Stein, J.A., & Nyamathi, A. (2000). Gender Differences in Behavioural and Psychosocial Predictors of HIV Testing and Return for Test Results in a High-risk Population. *AIDS Care*, Vol.12, No.3, (June 2000), pp.343-356, ISSN 1360-0451

Stolte, I.G., Gras, M., Van Benthem, B.H., Coutinho, R.A., & van den Hoek, J.A. (2003). HIV Testing Behaviour among Heterosexual Migrants in Amsterdam. *AIDS Care*, Vol. 15, No.4, (August 2003), pp. 563-574, ISSN 1360-0451

Stronks, K., Ravelli, C.J., & Reijneveld, A.S. (2001). Immigrants in the Netherlands: Equal Access for Equal Needs? *Journal of Epidemiology and Community Health*, Vol.55, No.10, (October 2001), pp. 701-707, ISSN 1470-2738

Ventura-Filipe, E.M., Bugamelli, L.E., Leme, B., Santos, N.J., Garcia, S., Paiva, V., & Hearst, N. (2000). Risk Perception and Counseling among HIV Positive Women in Sao Paulo, Brazil. *International Journal of STD and AIDS*, Vol.11, No.2, (February 2000), pp. 112–114, ISSN 1758-1052

Wang, B., Li, X., Stanton, B., & McGuire, J. (2010). Correlates of HIV/STD Testing and Willingness to Test among Rural-to-Urban Migrants in China. *AIDS and Behavior*, Vol.14, No.4, (August 2010), pp. 891-903, ISSN 1573-3254

WHO (2010). *Health of Migrants: The Way Forward - Report of a Global Consultation, Madrid, Spain, 3-5 March 2010*, WHO, ISBN 978 92 4 159950 4, Geneva, Switzerland

Wong, F., Campsmith, M., Nakamura, G., Crepaz, N., & Begley, E. (2004). HIV Testing and Awareness of Care-related Services among a Group of HIV-positive Asian Americans and Pacific Islanders in the United States: Findings from a Supplemental HIV/AIDS Surveillance Project. *AIDS Education and Prevention*, Vol.16, No.5, (October 2004), pp. 440–447, ISSN 1943-2755

Worthington, C., & Myers, T. (2003). Factors Underlying Anxiety in HIV Testing: Risk Perceptions, Stigma, and the Patient-provider Power Dynamic. *Qualitative Health Research*, Vol. 13, No.5, (May 2003), pp. 636–655, ISSN 1049-7323

7

Pediatric HIV Testing Challenges in Resource Limited Settings

Gumbo Felicity Zvanyadza
University of Zimbabwe/ College of Health Sciences
Zimbabwe

1. Introduction

According to UNAIDS, the joint United Nations Program on HIV/AIDS, 2.5 million children younger than 15 years are living with HIV, and during 2008 nearly half a million children were infected with HIV. Most of these children (67%) were from sub-Saharan Africa, and mother to child transmission was the major route of infection (91%) (Vermund 2004). HIV is one of the major causes of infant mortality in developing countries (Marston et al., 2005; Rashid et al., 2005). Prevention of mother to child transmission (PMTCT) of HIV has become an important cornerstone to reduce child mortality in sub-Saharan Africa. The research achievements in PMTCT are remarkable. Unfortunately, it has proved much more difficult to translate these findings into practice in resource-poor settings.

Virology tests are expensive and require sophisticated laboratory facilities. The expense of creating a laboratory with appropriate quality control and assurance to perform virology testing is significant, as well as the recurrent costs of test reagents. Laboratory technicians and scientists are in short supply in many resource-limited countries, and highly trained technicians may have high turnover because they are often sought by researchers and other countries. Venipuncture of infants requires training and supplies that are often unavailable outside large cities. Transport difficulties and distances may prohibit whole blood samples from reaching high-level laboratories in adequate time and condition for testing. Difficulties in returning results quickly to clinical sites may reduce acceptability of testing and cause results to go unclaimed. Effective infant diagnosis programs require a combination of clinical, serologic, and virologic approaches to the question of infant HIV status (Creek et al., 2007).

Diagnosis is an important aspect of providing treatment and care to those children infected. The earlier the diagnosis is made the better the outcome for patients. High mortality in the first few months of life has been reported particularly in resource limited settings (Zijenah et al., 1998, 2004). Approximately 20% can die by 6 months of life, 35-40% by 1 year of age and 50-60% by 2 years (Newell at al., 2004; Obimbo et al., 2004). Currently early detection is very possible with virologic assays which are sensitive and specific. Serologic methods such as HIV- Enzyme Linked Immunosorbent Assay (ELISA), Western blot, and Immunofluorescence Assay can be used to diagnose HIV infection in children older than 18 months. Cheaper rapid diagnostic tests have been introduced which can be used at the point of care (Brambilla et al., 2003).

2. HIV serology

Serology which is appropriate for diagnosing HIV infection in older children can not be used in young infants who are less than 18 months of age, particularly those breast feeding because of interference with maternal antibodies. Maternal antibodies cross the placenta so they can give false positive results in HIV uninfected children. The test does not distinguish maternal from infant antibodies (Lujan-Zilbermann et al., 2006). However when HIV antibodies are not present in HIV exposed children younger than 18 months but older than one year who are not breast feeding or in the window period, a diagnosis of HIV negative status can be made (Alecdort et al., as cited in Creek et al., 2007). Current assays have both a sensitivity and specificity greater than 99% in children older than 18 months. (Palasanthiran et al., 1994). If the initial serologic test is positive, a second ELISA or EIA is performed on the same specimen. If the second test is positive a confirmatory test is indicated, commonly an HIV-1 Western blot or an HIV-1 indirect immunofluorescence antibody assay (Brambillia et al., 2003). These gold standard tests are expensive and require a long waiting period before results can be obtained by clinicians in charge mainly because of the batching of specimens to save reagents.

Rapid tests have become important in resource limited settings mainly because of use by personnel with limited skills, ability to give out results immediately at site which makes counseling easier. Specificity and sensitivity is reasonable and comparable to those of EIAs used for screening (Mylonakis et al., 2000).

In young infants HIV rapid antibody tests can have a role if the maternal HIV infection status is unknown. HIV exposure can be confirmed with a positive result and excluded with a negative one. Infants lose maternal antibodies at different times, as a result young infants who have lost maternal antibodies can be presumed HIV negative at a younger age with rapid tests if they are not breast feeding and not in the window period. This is a reasonable low cost approach of ruling out HIV infection in HIV exposed infants. A large proportion of HIV uninfected children are seronegative by 9 months of age and some as early as 4 months (Blackburn et al., 2006). Errors have been found with some rapid test kits reporting false negative results particularly in severe illness which is associated with hypogammaglobulinaemia hence clinical judgment and appropriate physical examination is necessary at the diagnostic stage.

The testing of saliva for HIV antibody may be useful in infants because oral fluid contains lower concentrations of all antibodies in comparison with blood. Diminishing maternal HIV antibodies in HIV-exposed but uninfected infants likely become undetectable earlier in oral fluids than in blood. Laboratory-based or rapid HIV tests performed on oral fluid can potentially exclude HIV infection earlier in life, and sample collection is less traumatic for the infant and caregiver. Further validation of oral fluid assays is needed to establish the youngest age at which seroreversion can be detected and to determine the sensitivity and specificity of the test at different ages (Sherman et al 2005).

3. Virologic testing

Nucleic acid testing methods include HIV-1 Deoxyribonucleic acid polymerase chain reaction (DNA PCR), HIV Ribonucleic acid polymerase chain reaction (RNA PCR) and HIV-1 p24 Antigen. Polymerase chain reaction (PCR) assays detect HIV-1 DNA within peripheral blood mononuclear cells (PBMC). Proper specimen collection procedures and processing are important for the validity of the results. Whole blood should be collected in tubes containing edentate calcium disodium (EDTA) or acid citrate dextrose as anticoagulants (Brambilla et al., 2003). Major challenges faced here include the cost of bleeding the patient, namely syringes, needles and appropriate blood tubes. Transportation of specimens and storage are also important where frequent power cuts compromise the quality of results.

3.1 HIV deoxyribonucleic acid (DNA) PCR

HIV DNA PCR is the standard method for virologic diagnosis of HIV in infants in the developed world. It has been used for many years, is the diagnostic test of choice recommended by the WHO, and has acceptable sensitivity and specificity (Bremer et al., 1996; Sherman et al., 2005). For HIV -1 subtype B, the sensitivity and specificity of HIV-1 DNA PCR assays approach 96% and 99% respectively, by 28 days of age. They are less sensitive for detection of non-B subtype infection (Lujan-Zilbermann et al, 2006). HIV infection can often be detected at birth, and essentially all perinatal infections are detectable by 4 weeks of age (Sherman et al., 2004). Infections acquired postpartum (i.e., through breast-feeding) can be detected by 4-6 weeks after the last exposure. Different PCR tests exist world wide and not all tests are equally accurate with all HIV subtypes. The cost can range from $8 USD to $16USD per test (Creek et al., 2007).

3.2 Ribonucleic acid (RNA) PCR

An HIV RNA PCR, quantitative or qualitative, is also an accurate method of diagnosing HIV in young infants, with sensitivity and specificity comparable with DNA PCR testing. However, this test is more expensive and requires the use of plasma, which is difficult to obtain from infants and transport intact. HIV RNA PCR is routinely used to monitor disease progression and response to HAART. Whole blood specimens collected should be processed within 6 hours for accurate results which poses a challenge in resource poor settings (Brambilla et al 2003).

3.3 Real-time PCR

Real-time PCR allows the technician to view the increase in the amount of DNA or RNA when it is amplified. Real-time PCR as a new approach is gaining acceptability because of its improved rapidity, sensitivity, reproducibility, and the reduced risk of carry-over contamination, and it may reduce the cost of nucleic acid testing (Katsoulidou et al., 2006 & Zhao et al., 2002 as cited in Creek et al., 2007).This method is in use in numerous research settings and performs very well. However, at present the only commercial kits available are for quantitative and not qualitative detection of HIV, and large-scale use of these assays for public health programs has not been attempted (Creek et al., 2007).

3.4 Ultrasensitive (US) p24 antigen assay

The US p24 antigen assay is slightly less sensitive than HIV PCR in identifying HIV infection in infants across various subtypes and has a specificity similar to that of HIV PCR

(Patton et al., 2006; Sherman et al., 2004;) quantitative viral protein detection assay utilizes simpler technology than is required for detection of viral nucleic acids, but it is still relatively complex with multiple processing steps. US p24 is not in general use because studies validating it for infant diagnosis are recent, and achieving valid results in field settings has been challenging. US p24 may provide a useful alternative where PCR is not available. It can be used as a marker of disease progression and therapeutic response (Keenan et al., 2005).

3.5 Dried blood spots (DBS)

The HIV-1-DNA PCR on dried blood spots have made a significant difference in giving young HIV infected infants a chance for survival by early diagnosis. Spotting of whole blood onto filter paper offers technical and economic advantages over conventional venipuncture methods since it simplifies sample collection and transport to reference laboratories for diagnostic testing and viral load quantification (Zhang et al., 2002). Because infant blood for testing can be taken by simply pricking a heel, toe, or finger and dried cards are stable for relatively long periods without refrigeration; many logistical barriers to infant testing can be overcome using this simple technique. However proper training of staff is required to improve validity of results. PCR performed on DBS is as accurate as PCR performed on whole blood but has higher reagent cost and some increase in processing time. DNA and RNA PCR, both standard and real time, have been successfully performed on DBS in many settings and HIV subtypes with no loss of accuracy (Cassol et al., 1996; Lyamuya et al., 2000; Sherman et al., 2004; 19, 26-27). Routine collection of DBS for early infant diagnosis is being implemented in many countries. Dried blood spots have been successfully used to measure HIV-1 RNA in patients and to diagnose perinatal HIV infection. Some studies have reported low stability of nucleic acids in dried blood spots particularly when stored under inappropriate conditions.

Dried blood spots may also be used for HIV-1 sub typing and genotypic resistance testing (Fiscus et al., 2006). Although HIV-1 viral load can be successfully enumerated using dried blood spots there are limitations posed by volume of blood or plasma especially if sensitive nucleic acid testing is done or multiple tests are done on the same sample. The Vivest (formerly referred to as SampleTanker) is an economical dried specimen storage transportation system where significantly increased plasma volumes can be shipped at optimum temperatures (Zanoni et al., 2010). Its use was validated in Brazil, it was demonstrated that DNA HIV-1 viral load results from dried plasma eluted from Vivest are generally comparable to that of fresh plasma. Its use present a cost effective way of transporting specimens in resource poor settings where the logistics associated with shipping frozen plasma are expensive(Zanoni et al., 2010).

4. Conclusion

Clinicians looking after children should be aware of the different tests available to diagnose HIV infection in children which are useful in resource limited settings. All the different tests have different applications in these settings and accuracy should not be compromised so that the goal of reducing child mortality is met.

5. References

[1] Aledort JE, Ronald A, Le Blancq SM, et al. (March 2011). Reducing the burden of HIV/AIDS in infants: the contribution of improved diagnostics. 03.03.11, Available from http://www.nature.com/diagnostics

[2] Blackburn L, Sherman G, Coovadia A, et al. (2006). HIV rapid tests can be used as a screening tool to reduce HIV DNA PCR assays in a resource-poor setting. Presented at *the 2006 HIV/AIDS Implementers' Meeting*, 2006, Durban, South Africa.

[3] Brambilla D, Jennings C, Aldrovandi G, et al.(2003). Multicenter evaluation of use of dried blood and plasma spot specimens in quantitative assays for human immunodeficiency virus RNA: measurement, precision, and RNA stability. *Journal of Clinical Microbiology* vol 41, pp. 1888-93.

[4] Bremer JW, Lew JF, Cooper E, et al.(1996). Diagnosis of infection with human immunodeficiency virus type 1 by a DNA polymerase chain reaction assay among infants enrolled in the Women and Infants' Transmission Study. *Journal of Pediatrics* vol 129, pp. 198-207.

[5] Cassol S, Weniger BG, Babu PG, et al.(1996) Detection of HIV type 1 env subtypes A, B, C, and E in Asia using dried blood spots: a new surveillance tool for molecular epidemiology. *AIDS Res Hum Retroviruses* , vol 12, pp.1435-41.

[6] Creek TL, Sherman GG, Nkengasong J, et al. Infant human immunodeficiency virus diagnosis in resource limited settings: issues, technologies, and country experiences. American Journal of Obstetrics and Gynecology supplement 2007. O4.08.11. Available from http://wwwAJOG.com

[7] Fiscus S, Cheng B, Crowe SM, et al (2006). HIV-1 Viral Load Assays for Resource-Limited Settings. *Plos Medicine* .vol 3, No 10, pp. 1743-51

[8] Katsoulidou A, Petrodaskalaki M, Sypsa V, et al.(2006). Evaluation of the clinical sensitivity for the quantification of human immunodeficiency virus type 1 RNA in plasma: comparison of the new COBAS TaqMan HIV-1 with three current HIVRNA assays—LCx HIV RNA quantitative, VERSANT HIV-1 RNA 3.0 (bDNA) and COBAS AMPLICOR HIV-1 Monitor v1.5. *Journal of Virology Methods,* vol 131, pp. 168-74.

[9] Keenan PA, Keenan JM & Branson BM. (2005). Rapid HIV testing. Wait time reduced from days to minutes. *Postgrad Medicine,* vol 117, pp. 47-52

[10] Lujan-Zilbermann J, Rodriguez CA & Emmanuel PJ.(2006). Pediatric HIV Infection: Diagnostic Laboratory Methods. *Fetal and Pediatric Pathology* , vol 25, pp. 249-260

[11] Lyamuya E, Olausson-Hansson E, Albert J, et al. (2000). Evaluation of a prototype Amplicor PCR assay for detection of human immunodeficiency virus type 1 DNA in blood samples from Tanzanian adults infected with HIV-1 subtypes A, C and D. *Journal of Clinical Virology* , vol 17, pp. 57-63.

[12] Marston M, Zaba B, Solomon JA, et al.(2005). Estimating the net effect of HIV on child mortality in African populations affected by generalized HIV epidemics. *Journal of Acquired Immune Deficiency Syndrome* , vol 38, No 2, pp. 219-227

[13] Mylonakis E, Paliou M, Lally M, et al. (2000). . Laboratory testing for infection with the human immunodeficiency virus: Established and novel approaches. *American Journal of Medicine* , vol 109, pp. 568-576

[14] Newell ML, Coovadia H, Cortina-Borja M, et al. (2004). Mortality of infected and uninfected infants born to HIV-infected mothers in Africa: a pooled analysis. *Lancet,* vol 364, pp. 1236-43.

[15] Obimbo EM, Mbori-Ngacha DA, Ochien JO, et al. (2004). Predictors of early mortality in a cohort of human immunodeficiency virus type 1-infected African children. *Pediatrics Infectious Disease Journal* , vol 23, pp. 536-43.

[16] Palasanthiran P, Robertson P, Graham GG, et al .(1994). Decay of transplacental human immunodeficiency virus type-1 (HIV-1) antibodies in neonates and infants. *Annu Conf Australas Soc HIV Med* , vol 6, No 165 (abstract)

[17] Patton JC, Sherman GG, Coovadia AH, et al. (2006). Ultrasensitive human immunodeficiency virus type 1 p24 antigen assay modified for use on dried whole-blood spots as a reliable, affordable test for infant diagnosis. Clinical Vaccine Immunology, vol 13, pp. 152-5.

[18] Sherman GG & Jones SA.(2005). Oral fluid human immunodeficiency virus tests: improved access to diagnosis for infants in poorly resourced prevention of mother to child transmission programs *Pediatrics Infectious Disease Journal* , vol 24, pp. 253-6

[19] Sherman GG, Cooper PA, Coovadia AH, et al.(2005). Polymerase chain reaction for diagnosis of human immunodeficiency virus infection in infancy in low resource settings. *Pediatrics Infectious Disease Journal* , *vol* 24, pp. 993-7.

[20] Sherman GG, Jones SA, Coovadia AH, et al..(2004). PMTCT from research to reality—results from a routine service. *South African Medical Journal,* vol 94, pp. 289-92.

[21] Sherman GG, Stevens G & Stevens WS. (2004). Affordable diagnosis of human immunodeficiency virus infection in infants by p24 antigen detection. *Pediatrics Infectious Disease Journal* , vol 23, pp. 173-6.

[22] Vermund SH.(2004). Prevention of mother to child transmission of HIV infection in Africa. *Tropical HIV Medicine,* vol 12, No 5, pp. 130-134

[23] Zanoni M, Cortes R, Diaz RS, et al. (2010). Comparative effectiveness of dried plasma HIV-1 viral load testing in Brazil using ViveST for sample collection. *Journal of clinical virology,* vol. 49, No 4, pp. 245-248

[24] Zhang M & Versalovic J.(2002). HIV update: diagnostic tests and markers of disease progression and response to therapy. *American Journal of Clinical Pathology,* vol 18(suppl) pp. S26-S32

[25] Zhao Y, Yu M, Miller JW, et al. Quantification of human immunodeficiency virus type 1 proviral DNA by using TaqMan technology. *Journal of Clinical Microbiology,* vol 40, pp. 675-8.

[26] Zijenah LS, Moulton LH, Illiff P, et al. (2004). Timing of mother to child transmission of HIV 1 and infant mortality in the first 6 months of life in Harare, Zimbabwe. *AIDS,* vol 18, No 2, pp. 273-280

[27] Zijenah L, Mbizvo MT, Kasule J, et al.(1998). Mortality in the first two years among infants born to HIV-infected women in Harare. *Journal of Infectious Diseases,* vol 178, pp. 109-113

8

HIV Drug Resistance in Sub-Saharan Africa – Implications for Testing and Treatment

Kuan-Hsiang Gary Huang[1,3], Helen Fryer[1], Dominique Goedhals[2,3], Cloete van Vuuren[2,3] and John Frater[1,3]
[1]*University of Oxford, Oxford,*
[2]*University of Free State, Bloemfontein,*
[3]*Bloemfontein-Oxford Collaborative Group*
[1,3]*UK*
[2,3]*South Africa*

1. Introduction

This chapter will review the current evidence surrounding the emergence of HIV drug resistance in sub-Saharan Africa, the current guidelines for the drug resistance testing, and their implication. Data from a cohort study in the Free State province of South Africa will be used as an applied example in the discussion.

2. ARV and mechanism of drug resistance emergence

The first antiretroviral therapy (ARV) drug, azidothymidine (zidovudine, originally developed to treat cancer), was discovered to inhibit the reverse transcriptase (RT) enzyme of HIV in 1986 (Yarchoan, et al. 1986). Since then, more inhibitor classes to other essential steps of viral replication have been discovered (Barbaro, et al. 2005). The ability of HIV to mutate and recombine frequently allows it to evade individual ARV rapidly (Aboulker and Swart 1993). In 1996, the introduction of combination ARV, often termed highly active antiretroviral therapy (HAART), introduced a dramatic treatment response to patients. HAART delays disease progression, reduces AIDS mortality (by up to 70% annually) and partially restores CD4 T cells, but cannot clear HIV infection (Palella, et al. 1998). Furthermore, HAART delays the emergence of resistant HIV isolates, which accumulated rapidly during the pre-HAART era, when mono-, or dual-, therapy were in use (Kuritzkes 2007).

Under multiple ARV drug selection (usually 3 agents, balancing clinical efficacy and patient tolerability), HIV is successfully suppressed (Larder, et al. 1995). However, given time or opportunity (such as when therapy is interrupted or not adhered to), HIV can acquire resistance to one or more agents in HAART regimens, requiring changing of failed ARV components. Drug toxicity is another major health concern (Carvajal-Rodriguez, et al. 2007, Larder, et al. 1993, Larder, et al. 1995). Although some drug escape mutants are impaired in replication fitness, others seem unaffected or may even have increased fitness (Armstrong, et al. 2009, Garcia-Lerma, et al. 2004, Prado, et al. 2002). Similar to escape seen in natural selection, reversion to wild type virus occurs rapidly following treatment cessation. Drug compensatory mutations also arise secondarily to restore fitness in the mutants harbouring costly escape (Gandhi, et al. 2003, Stanford University 2011).

Furthermore, intra-subtype and inter-subtype differences in HIV genetic sequences evoke different pathways leading to escape (Pieniazek, et al. 2000). Therefore, concerted efforts, surveillance programs and comprehensive databases have been set up to describe subtype-specific drug resistance mutations and their accessory mutations (which may either have predisposing, compensating or augmenting effects to drug concurrent resistance mutations) (Bennett, et al. 2009, Gifford, et al. 2007, Stanford University 2011).

2.1 HIV, HAART and drug resistance in sub-Saharan Africa

In sub-Saharan Africa, 22.5 million people (5% of adult population) are infected with HIV, effectively harbouring over two thirds of the world prevalence (33.3 million) (UNAIDS/WHO 2011). Furthermore, in 2009, HIV infected over 1.8 million adults and children in the sub-Saharan region, and caused 1.3 million deaths through AIDS. This represents public health emergency, requiring immediate effective intervention. However, resource limitation, escalating disease burden and established stigmata remain major challenges to effective intervention. In particular, poverty and resource limitations undermine HIV control by constraining the access, availability and affordability of HIV testing, anti-retroviral therapy (ARV), follow up, and skilled staff (UNAIDS/WHO 2011).

Similarly, sub-Saharan African nations lacked the resources to research and develop their own ARV and HAART. Fortunately, although the ARV and HAART regimens were originally designed to inhibit subtype B HIV-1, they are also efficacious against other subtypes, including C - the dominant subtype infecting sub-Saharan Africa (Frater, et al. 2001, Gordon, et al. 2003, Kantor, et al. 2005). In the *pol* gene subtype C varies from subtype B by 10-12% at the nucleotide level, yet these genotypic differences do not appear to confer major pre-therapy drug resistance, although may be associated with more accessory resistance mutations and different molecular pathways to resistance (Frater, et al. 2002, Gordon, et al. 2003, Pieniazek, et al. 2000, Robertson, et al. 2000, Sanches, et al. 2007, Velazquez-Campoy, et al. 2001).

As HAART became available, many sub-Saharan Africa states initiated large scale primary care dispensing of HAART to qualifying patients according to the CDC and WHO guidelines (Department of Health 2003). However, the regional circulating strains of HIV remain poorly characterised in their molecular epidemiology and genotypic profiles. In addition, various mono- and dual-ARV are also indicated in the prevention of mother-to-child transmission (PMTCT) program of different sub-Saharan regions, exposing patients to potential resistance development (Jourdain, et al. 2004). Therefore, ahead of the mass dispensing of HAART, it is important to study the molecular characterisation and baseline pre-therapy drug resistance profiles of subtype C HIV-1 in South Africa (Department of Health 2003, Gilks, et al. 2006). This will also contribute to the long-term follow up of resistance development.

2.2 Characterising drug resistance

There are three types of ARV resistance (DHHS-Panel 2011):

- Clinical resistance: occurs when viral replication continues despite HAART institution, and carries direct clinical impact. Clinical criteria exist to define virological (increase viral load, VL) and immunological failure (poor increase or decreasing of CD4 cell count and development of opportunistic infection) during HAART.

- Phenotypic resistance: can assess viral growth in the presence of ARV *in vitro*. This test is highly specialized (requiring recombination of HIV *pol* gene with a laboratory viral backbone) and is time consuming (viral culture and measurements take three to four weeks). The test is more expensive, and has no proven advantage over genotypic resistance testing, and may suffer reduced sensitivity in the detection of minority resistant mutant isolates (when the mutants are present at less than 20% of circulating viral population).
- Genotypic resistance: is conducted to sequence the *RT* and *protease* genes for the detection of known resistance mutations (*Integrase* sequencing can also be done, on request). The test is considerably less expensive, time consuming and more widely available when compared to the phenotypic resistance assay (although the level of expertise required is still very high and not common to routine diagnostic laboratories). Furthermore, different sequencing assay techniques could be employed to improve sensitivity of detecting minority resistant mutants. A 'virtual phenotype' can also be imputed to measure the phenotypic impact of a mutation using laboratory strain manipulation. To date, global databases including Stanford HIV drug resistance database (Stanford HIV db) have collated, analysed and summarised considerable amounts of different genotype-treatment, genotype-clinical, and genotype-phenotype evidence based academic publications.

The identification of drug resistance in sub-Saharan Africa has become a major issue in patients receiving HAART and in drug-naïve individuals (Shekelle, et al. 2007). Guidelines exist for the surveillance of both - the World Health Organisation (WHO) and Stanford HIV db publish a list of mutations for use in surveillance of transmitted drug resistance (TDRM) and the International AIDS Society (IAS) produce a list for use in the monitoring of treated populations (HRDS-Team 2003, Johnson, et al. 2008, Stanford University 2011). The WHO, Stanford HIV db and IAS committees regularly update the definitions and clinical significance (phenotypic resistance, clinical association and outcome meta-analyses) of drug resistance mutations and drug associated polymorphisms (Bennett, et al. 2009, Shafer, et al. 2007). However, authorities disagree on the classification of naturally occurring non-clade B polymorphisms, drug-associated polymorphisms not associated with direct measurable drug resistances, and polymorphisms associated with reversion of previous drug-resistance mutation (Stanford University 2011). Therefore, many of the Stanford db's 'potentially low grade' and 'low grade' resistance mutations are excluded from the IAS and WHO surveillance lists, showing there are discrepancies between the key opinion leaders. Recently, the updated TDRM list from the Stanford HIV db has become unified with the WHO guidelines (Gilks, et al. 2006, HRDS-Team 2003). The mutations in the TDRM surveillance list are selected on the basis that they are non-polymorphic, clinically significant and applicable across all subtypes. The implementation of such a standard should facilitate a specific method to assess changes in drug resistance prevalence in populations over time (Garcia-Diaz, et al. 2008, HRDS-Team 2003, Seebregts, et al. 5-8 June 2007). It is clearly ideal to have a single mutations list to screen all populations, however the possibility exists that for South Africa where the dynamics of therapy provision and the more recent introduction of universal access to HAART makes for a unique situation, a subtype C-specific list may become more applicable (SATuRN-Database, et al. 2011).

3. Molecular epidemiology and genotypic drug resistance in treatment-naïve HIV population of South Africa

In South Africa (SA, Figure 1), 5.5 million people are infected with HIV (ASSA 2007, UNAIDS/WHO 2011, Venter 2005). Since 2004, the SA government has made antiretroviral therapy (ARV) available to HIV positive individuals through public sector ARV programs - an initiative with significant clinical, public health and economic impact (Department of Health 2003, Egger, et al. 1997, Frater 2002, Palella, et al. 1998, Sow, et al. 2007, Venter 2005).

Until recently, only a few small to medium-sized South African cohorts have reported the molecular characterisation and baseline pre-therapy resistance profiles of HIV infection, predominantly amongst the KwaZulu Natal, Gauteng and Limpopo provinces (Bessong, et al. 2006, Gordon, et al. 2003, Pillay, et al. 2002, Shekelle, et al. 2007). There are also emerging data on drug resistance from other major cities of sub-Saharan countries such as Uganda, Tanzania, Botswana, Zimbabwe, Zambia, Malawi and Kenya (Bussmann, et al. 2005, Eshleman, et al. 2009, Gordon, et al. 2003, Hamers, et al. 2010, Kamoto and Aberle-Grasse 2008, Lihana, et al. 2009, Mosha, et al. 2011, SATuRN-Database, et al. 2011, Shekelle, et al. 2007, Tshabalala, et al. 2011). There is currently no similar information available from other less urbanised regions of South Africa, such as Free State Province (Figure 1) with a population of approximately 3 million, an antenatal clinic HIV prevalence of 33.9%, and the life expectancy estimate of 46.5 years (ASSA 2007). Under the Free State Comprehensive Care, Management and Treatment of HIV and AIDS program, highly active antiretroviral therapy (HAART) has been available since 2004 as a combination stavudine and lamivudine with either nevirapine or Kaletra, and has significantly reduced the number of HIV-related deaths (hazard ratio 0.14) (Fairall, et al. 2008).

In patients who report that they are drug-naive, resistance mutations might either reveal transmitted variants or might indicate that patients are not, in fact, drug-naive or are unaware of previous ARV exposure (Garcia-Diaz, et al. 2008). The extent to which unrecognized access contributes to the level of resistance in patients enrolling onto public sector ARV is unknown in South Africa, and very difficult to measure. Prior to the introduction of the public sector ARV treatment programme, ARV drugs were available for the PMTCT through private clinics and other unregulated routes, although previous studies suggest a low prevalence of baseline drug resistance in South Africa (Bessong, et al. 2006, Gordon, et al. 2003, Pillay, et al. 2002, Shekelle, et al. 2007).

Here, the discussion on molecular epidemiology and pre-therapy drug resistance will be applied to a South African clinical cohort study (Huang, et al. 2009). In the Free State province of South Africa, 425 HIV type-1 (HIV-1)-positive patients newly recruited to the public sector ARV treatment programme and reporting to be drug-naïve were studied. The molecular epidemiology of HIV-1 infection within this region were characterised, and the prevalence of drug resistance and other polymorphisms associated with drug exposure were measured. A correlation existed between low CD4 T cell counts and drug-selected polymorphisms, suggesting that many mutations in drug-naive individuals are not transmitted, but are the result of acquired resistance through unrecognised ARV access.

The aims of this study were: to describe the viral molecular epidemiology of Free State Province, South Africa (Figure 1), to investigate the prevalence of drug-resistance associated mutations, and resistance to HAART in the pre-therapy cohort and to model the impact of ART availability on baseline antiretroviral resistance.

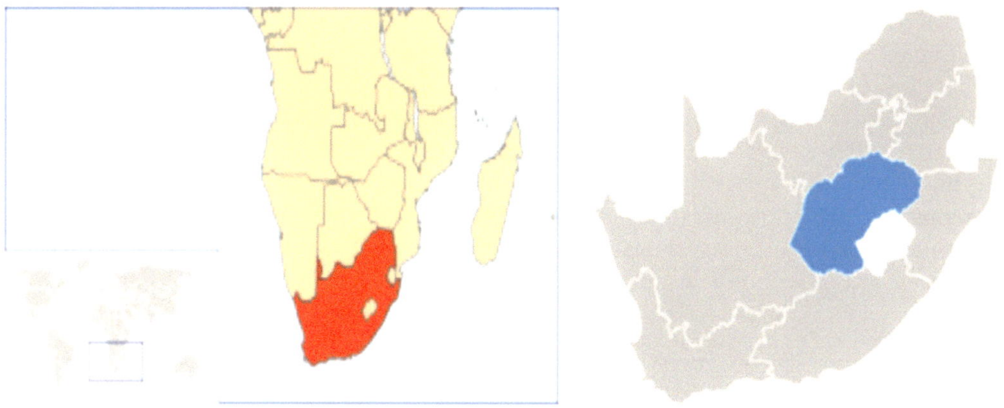

Left panel: South Africa (in red) at the south of Sub-Saharan Africa (boxed and enlarged from the world map in left lower corner).
Right panel: Free State province (in blue, capital: Bloemfontein) and KwaZulu Natal province (in purple, capital: Durban) are two of the nine provinces in central east region of South Africa.

Fig. 1. Map of South Africa and its provinces, figure modified from original (Wikimedia-Commons 2010)

4. Experimental approach to the Free State cohort

In total, 884 adult patients were recruited at their first visit to government antiretroviral therapy (ART) clinics in the Free State province of South Africa between February and September 2006. Informed consent for additional sampling of plasma for viral sequencing was obtained. All patients had been diagnosed with HIV infection at local primary care clinics, and then referred to district or regional HIV clinics to be assessed for suitability for HAART. On attending the clinic, patients were counseled by trained HIV nurses and asked directly whether they had previously received PMTCT, mono-, dual- or triple antiretroviral therapy. Patients who admitted previous drug exposure were excluded from this analysis. Demographic details, routine CD4 T cell counts and an additional 10ml of peripheral venous blood were collected from each individual patient. The ethics and study design were approved by the regional university and department of health.

The 884 patients were stratified according to their CD4 cell count into 5 groups as follows: <100 cells/μl (n = 195, 22.1%); 100-199 cells/μl (n= 212, 24%); 200-349 cells/μl (n=244, 27.6%); 350-499 cells/μl (n=123, 13.9%) and >500 cells/μl (n=110, 12.4%) (Table 1). From this cohort of 884, viral sequences were analysed from 425 patients to form the 'low' (<100 CD4 cells/μl; n=195), 'intermediate' (200-349 CD4 cells/μl; n=120) and 'high' (>500 CD4 cells/μl; n=110) CD4 cell count stratification groups.

For sequencing, RNA was extracted from plasma, converted to cDNA and then amplified by polymerase chain reaction before sequencing using ABI Big Dye terminator kits (Applied Biosystems). The primers used for the PCR and sequencing are described elsewhere (Frater, et al. 2007). From the 425 patients, complete *protease* sequences (99 amino acids) and amino acids 1-530 of *reverse transcriptase (RT)* were successfully. The *pol* gene sequences were submitted to the BioAfrica database and REGA HIV-1 subtype tool for subtype (www.bioafrica.net/subtypetool/html/) and locus identification (de Oliveira and Cassol

2011, de Oliveira, et al. 2005). Phylogenetic analysis and maximum likelihood trees were constructed using the General Time Reversible substitution model with optimised proportions of invariable sites and gamma distribution (GTR+G+I) using PAUP* (version 4.0 beta) and PhyML (version 2.4.4) software. The *pol* sequences of the cohort were compared to 986 well-characterised isolates from the BioAfrica database and those available on the Los Alamos database (www.hiv.lanl.gov) to determine subtype and lineage relationships (Guindon and Gascuel 2003, Los Alamos National Laboratory 2011). The Slatkin and Maddison test was used to assess clustering between the Free State Province sequences and other South African sequences, using MacClade (version 4) (Gifford, et al. 2007).

The *protease* and *RT* sequences were submitted to the Stanford drug resistance database (version 4.3.1, http://hivdb.stanford.edu/pages/algs/HIVdb.html) to identify subtype-associated polymorphisms and drug resistance mutations (Bennett, et al. 2008). The Stanford mutation scoring system (Table 1) was used to distinguish accessory mutations (mutation score 0-9) from clinically significant mutations ('potentially low level' resistance (score 10-14), 'low level' (score 15-30), 'intermediate level' (score 30-59) and 'high level' (score >=60) resistance) (Bennett, et al. 2008, Stanford University 2011).

An ordinary differential equation model was devised for this study to describe the dynamics of resistance to a single drug, such as Nevirapine, with a simple genetic resistance profile. The model encapsulates four main processes: selection of drug resistance in hosts treated in the public sector ARV treatment program, selection of drug resistance prior to 'official' treatment by other means such as private prescriptions, transmission of drug resistant strains to new hosts, and reversion to drug-sensitive strains in untreated hosts. Fisher's exact test (two tailed) and chi-square test were used to compare pre-therapy resistance findings between groups with different CD4 cell counts.

5. Molecular epidemiology and drug resistance prevalence in the Free State

In the analysis, there were three key findings. Firstly, there was evidence of multiple introductions of HIV-1 into the Free State, but random distribution of drug resistance-associated polymorphisms. Secondly, the overall prevalence of pre-therapy drug resistance was low, but drug-selected polymorphisms were concentrated among patients with low CD4 T cell counts. Thirdly, mathematical modelling suggested that baseline drug resistance may be driven by exposure to ARVs available through non-governmental routes and that, unless drug availability is controlled, resistance prevalence is likely to rise. In the section below, each of the findings will be described and discussed in more details.

5.1 Characterisation of the Free State province cohort in South African

Table 1 summarises the cohort demography and division for sub-studies. Patients attending antiretroviral clinics in Free State province during 2006 demonstrated a mean CD4 T cell count of 271 cells/µl, with 44.8% of patients possessing a CD4 cell counts of less than 200 cells/µl, significantly lower than other published chronic HIV cohorts (Kiepiela, et al. 2004). In an earlier study of 2777 chronically HIV infected individuals in the Pelonomi Hospital, Bloemfontein recruited between 1991 and 1997 (van der Ryst, et al. 1998), the mean CD4 T cell counts was 421 cells/µl. The low mean CD4 T cell counts seen in the Free State Cohort is likely

Category	Complete cohort	CD4⁺ T-cell count <100 cells/µl	100–199 cells/µl	200–349 cells/µl	350–499 cells/µl	≥500 cells/µl	*P*-value (χ^2 test for trend)
Patients in cohort, *n* (%)	884	195 (22.1)	212 (24.0)	244 (27.6)	123 (13.9)	110 (12.4)	–
Patients sampled, *n*	425	195	–	120	–	110	–
Patients with both protease and RT gene sequences, *n*	390	192	–	112	–	86	–
Mean age, years (±SD)	36.1 (9.1)	38 (8.9)	–	35.4 (9.0)	–	34.2 (9.2)	–
Mean CD4⁺ T-cell count, cells/µl (±SD)	271.3 (200.82)	45.36 (28.66)	–	269.96 (40.86)	–	651.80 (178.91)	–
Patients with drug resistance mutations, *n* (%)[a]	9 (2.3)	7 (3.6)	–	1 (0.9)	–	1 (1.2)	0.134 (0.055)
Total drug resistance mutations, *n*	11	9	–	1	–	1	–
Patients with non-accessory drug-associated mutations, *n* (%)[b]	16 (4.1)	13 (6.8)	–	2 (1.8)	–	1 (1.2)	0.015 (0.004)
Total non-accessory drug-associated mutations, *n*	19	16	–	2	–	1	–
Patients with any polymorphism at drug resistance-associated sites, *n* (%)[b]	64 (16.4)	37 (19.3)	–	15 (13.4)	–	12 (14.0)	0.193 (0.099)
Total naturally occurring drug-associated mutations, *n*	73	44	–	15	–	–	–

All patients listed in this table were infected with HIV type-1 (HIV-1) subtype C. Patients were stratified into three discrete groups according to baseline CD4⁺ T-cell count. Patients not falling into these groups were not analysed. The total number of mutations are also shown because some sequences contained more than one mutation. [a]Defined by the International AIDS Society–USA Drug Resistance Mutation list. [b]Defined by Stanford Drug Resistance Database.

Table 1. Details of HIV-1 positive patients recruited to three subgroups according to CD4 T cell count

a result of the cohort studied - ARV clinics tend to be enriched with patients presented during symptomatic phase of late HIV. There was no public ARV program available during 1990s. The availability of HAART from the government is expected to improve quality of life and reverse this population-wide fall in CD4 cell counts (Venter 2005).

The 884 patients were stratified according to CD4 T cell count, and viral sequences were analysed from 425 patients to form the low (<100 cells/μl; n=195), intermediate (200–349 cells/μl; n=120) and high (>500 cells/μl; n=110) CD4 T cell counts stratification groups. The mean CD4 T cell counts for all patients within the low, intermediate and high groups were 45.4, 270.0 and 651.8 cells/μl, respectively. The mean age of the cohort was 36.1 years (Table 1). Complete *protease* gene sequences (99 amino acids) and amino acids 1–530 of the *RT* gene were successfully amplified from 390 and 397 patients, respectively. The REGA subtyping tool revealed all isolates to be subtype C. All sequences were combined with reference sequences from the BioAfrica database and their phylogeny analysed using maximal likelihood trees (de Oliveira and Cassol 2011, de Oliveira, et al. 2005).

5.2 Molecular epidemiology studies revealed dynamic relationships between the local circulating viral isolates and the Southern Africa strains

The Free State is located in central South Africa and is relatively isolated from other South African centres. The phylogenetic analysis confirmed that Free State province is dominated by HIV-1 subtype C infection, much like the rest of South Africa (Table 1). There were multiple small but distinct clusters within the Free State, which suggests the mixing of HIV-1 strains from across South Africa, with migration into and through the Free State, possibly a result of the mining industry, transport routes and other economic reasons (Figure 2 and 3). However, despite these clusters, viruses with drug-resistance associated mutations are distributed randomly, suggesting that they have evolved recently as a result of individual drug exposure rather than being a transmission cluster.

In Figure 2, the maximum likelihood tree shows 390 HIV-1 *pol* sequences from the Free State in the context of local and global HIV-1 subtype C viruses from the BioAfrica database. The Free State strains (n=390) are in red, the South African strains (n=428) are in green, and remaining global subtype C strains (n=551) are in black. In Figure 3, the tree shows the phylogeny of the Free State patients (n=390) in the context of local HIV-1 subtype C virus strains from other provinces within SA (n=428). The Free State strains are highlighted in red, the drug resistant strains are highlighted in blue, whilst the SA reference strains (mainly from Gauteng, Kwa-Zulu Natal and Western Cape Province) are highlighted in green.

The Free State sequences appear to be distributed randomly amongst both Southern African (Figure 2) and South African (Figure 3) reference sequences. Quantitative analysis of clustering showed that 52.5% of sequences occurred in 61 clusters of between 2 and 18 sequences (mean 3.4 patients per cluster: 27 clusters of two, 10 clusters of three, 8 clusters of four, 3 clusters of five, 1 clusters of six, 2 clusters of seven, and 3 individual clusters of eight, nine and eighteen sequences). The analysis also shows that 70.6% of the Free State sequences (in isolation or in clusters) have a South African reference sequence as the nearest neighbour, but there is also clustering of sequences sampled from the Free State compared with other major South African centres (Slatkins and Maddison test, $P<0.001$). In addition, 96.1% of Free State strains are most closely related to a Southern African sequence and 97.2%

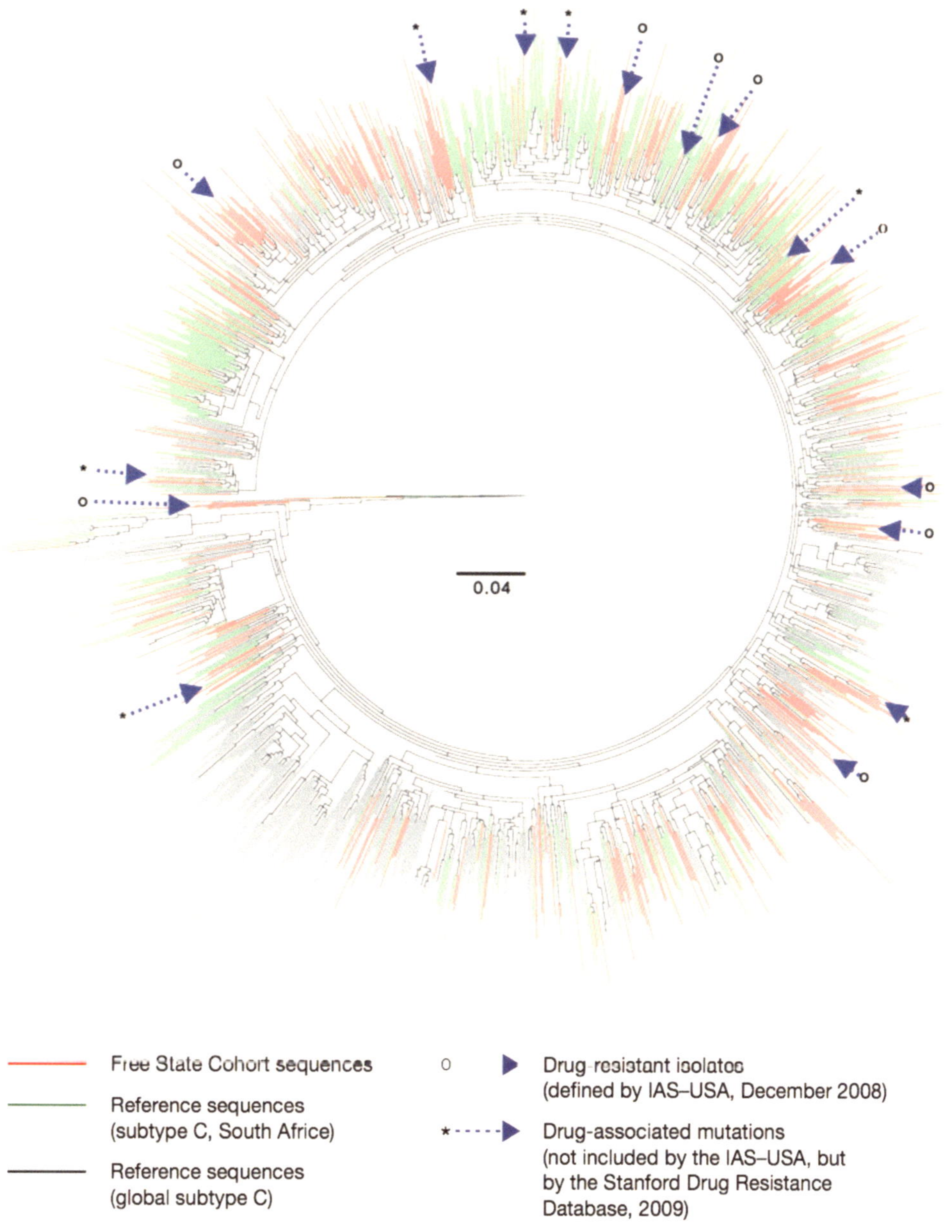

The *pol* gene of HIV-1 isolates sampled from Free State patients (red) are shown in the context of published South African (green) and non-South African (black) HIV-1 subtype C reference sequences. Resistant isolates defined by International AIDS Society (IAS)–USA and other drug-associated mutations defined by the Stanford Drug Resistance Database are shown (blue dotted arrows, ending in "o" and "*", respectively). This maximal likelihood tree was constructed using the general time reversible substitution model with optimised proportions of invariable sites and gamma distribution (GTR+G+I) using PAUP* (version 4.0 beta) and PhyML (version 2.4.4) software.

Fig. 2. Phylogenetic tree of the HIV-1 molecular epidemiology in the Free State, South Africa in the context of global HIV-1 subtype C *pol* reference sequences

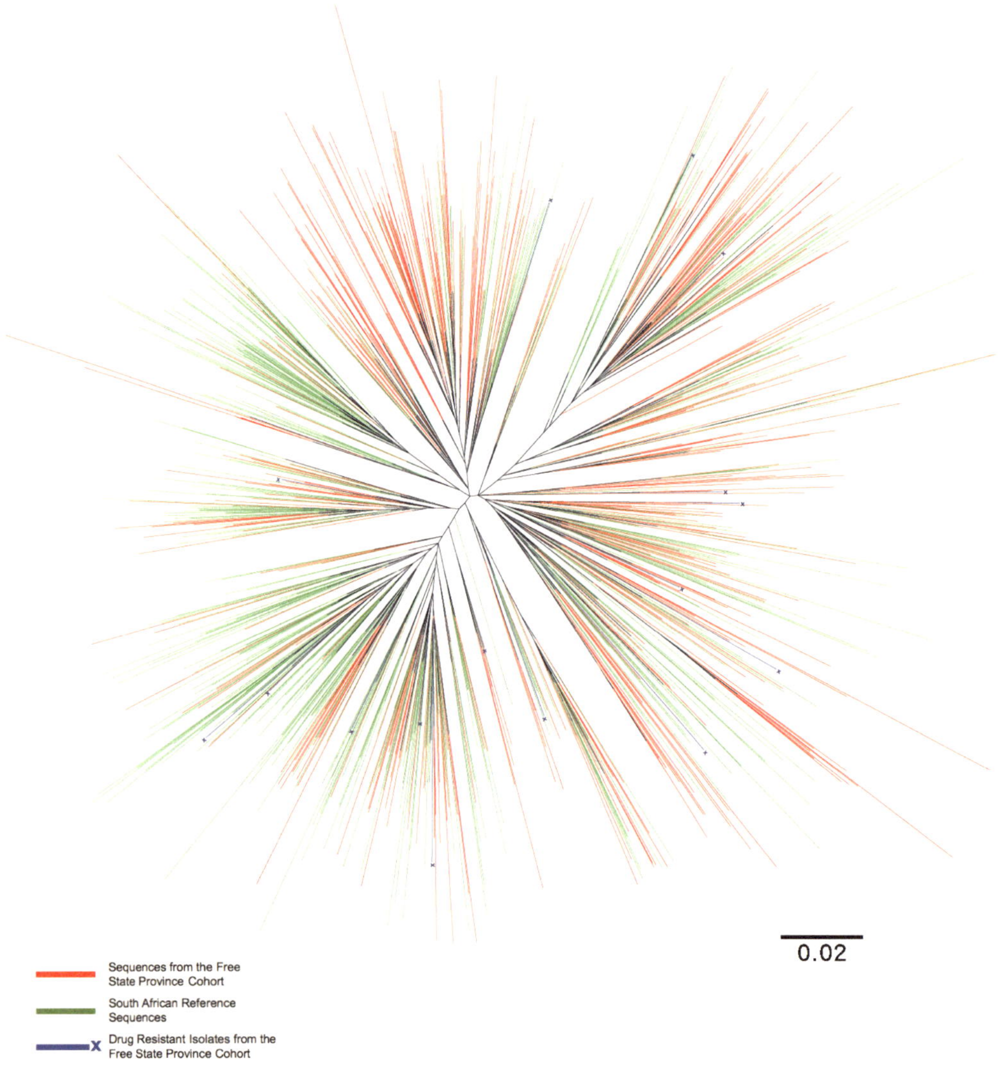

The *pol* gene of HIV isolates sampled from the Free State patients (in red) are shown in the context of published South African HIV-1 Subtype C database (in green). The two HIV population sequences showed remarkable homology, sharing common internal nodes. Only 1 group of 18 Free State isolates clustered with more than 10 sequences. The drug resistant isolates from Free State patients (blue stars) distribute sporadically across the tree. This maximal likelihood tree was constructed using the general time reversible substitution model with optimised proportions of invariable sites and gamma distribution (GTR+G+I) using PAUP* (version 4.0 beta) and PhyML (version 2.4.4) software.

Fig. 3. Phylogenetic tree describing HIV molecular epidemiology of the Free State Province and its drug resistant subjects in the context of South African HIV-1 subtype C reference sequences

of Free State strains are most closely related to an African sequence. Only 2.8% of the Free State sequences are closely related to a non-African sequence.

Sequences that contained any drug-associated polymorphism or a mutation from the IAS-USA surveillance list are indicated and are randomly distributed (Johnson, et al. 2008). The absence of linkage of these variant sequences does not support significant transmission of drug resistance within this cohort (Slatkins and Maddison test, P=0.85).

It is also important to note that in contrast to the developed nations, HIV molecular epidemiology remains poorly characterised in the sub-Saharan Africa. In an effort to fight the pandemic in its epicentre, initiatives have begun to enhance the understanding of molecular epidemiology of HIV infection in sub-Saharan African. Consortiums such as Southern African Treatment and Resistance Network (SATuRN) were established as a regional mirror of the Stanford HIV db in sub-Saharan region (SATuRN-Database, et al. 2011). In 2009, only 428 RT sequences were enlisted, with the active contribution from the likes of this cohort (n=390), the sample size of SATuRN is expanding rapidly.

5.3 Low prevalence of pre-therapy drug resistance in the Free State

All available pre-therapy *pol* gene sequences (n=390 for PR; n=397 for *RT* amino acids 1-530) from the Free State cohort were submitted to the Stanford HIV Resistance Database for identification of polymorphic sites associated with drug resistance. Although all potential resistance mutations were identified, specific attention was paid to the mutations from three drug classes currently being provided as part of the Free State public HAART regimen, namely protease inhibitor (PI), nucleoside reverse transcriptase inhibitor (NRTI), and non-nucleoside reverse transcriptase inhibitor (NNRTI).

According to the Stanford Drug Resistance Database list, the prevalence of non-accessory mutations was 4.1%, comprising 16 patients carrying a total of 19 non-accessory mutations (Table 1, Accessory mutations are defined as "atypical mutations or subtype-associated polymorphisms possibly related to secondary drug resistance" (Stanford University 2011)). The overall prevalence of clinically significant drug resistance mutations (according to the IAS–USA classification) was low (2.3%, Table 1), in concordence with the findings of previous smaller studies from South Africa (Bessong, et al. 2006, Gordon, et al. 2003, Johnson, et al. 2008, Pillay, et al. 2002, Shekelle, et al. 2007). A total of 64 (16.4%) patients sampled had a mutation at any of the drug resistance amino acid sites, including those that have been found to be naturally occurring polymorphisms (Table 1).

The 16 patients with non-accessory mutations - according to the Stanford definition - are detailed in Table 2. Of these, nine had clinically significant mutations according to the IAS-USA list. These were Y181C (n=2), K103N (n=3), Y188L (n=1), V106M (n=1), V108I (n=1) and K219E (n=1) in the *RT* gene, and M46L (n=1) and N88S (n=1) in the *protease* gene. The referral centres and local clinics where these patients had been recruited were either visited or contacted; however, in all but five cases the patients had been lost to follow-up. Of the four who had maintained undetectable viral loads on therapy, none had clinically significant IAS-USA defined mutations at baseline (V179D, M46L, A98G and T69N). The one patient identified with a detectable viral load on ARVs (13,000 RNA copies/ml after 5 months) had V179D at baseline, although no sequence data was available from subsequent samples to determine the development of resistance (Table 2). Of the 16 patients with significant resistance, 6 were male. Of the 10 females, the median age was 34.5 years (range 25–56).

Patient identification	Gender	Age, years	CD4+ T-cell count, cells/μl	PI major mutation (grade of resistance)[a]	NRTI mutation (grade of resistance)[a]	NNRTI mutation (grade of resistance)[a]	Response to therapy
OX2032	F	35	1	–	–	E138K (potentially low) and Y181C (high)	Lost to follow-up
OX428	M	37	2	–	–	A98G (potentially low)	Lost to follow-up
OX927	F	25	3	–	K219E (low)	Y181C (high)	Lost to follow-up
OX195	M	41	5	–	T69N (potentially low)	–	Lost to follow-up
OX693	M	31	14	–	–	V179D (potentially low)	VL=13,000 copies/ml 5 months after starting therapy
OX1	F	42	23	–	–	K103N (high)	Lost to follow-up
OX613	F	24	28	–	–	V179D (potentially low)	VL<25 copies/ml 28 months after starting 3TC/d4T/EFV
OX1082	M	37	30	–	–	V106M and Y188I (both high)	Lost to follow-up
OX2233	F	28	42	–	–	K103N (high)	Lost to follow-up
OX677	F	31	60	M46L (low)	–	–	VL<25 copies/ml 23 months after starting 3TC/d4T/EFV
OX2011	M	37	63	–	–	A98G (potentially low)	VL<25 copies/ml 33 months after starting 3TC/d4T/EFV
OX5	F	56	64	–	T69N (potentially low)	–	VL<25 copies/ml 36 months after starting 3TC/d4T/EFV
OX1006	M	43	64	–	–	V108I (potentially low)	Lost to follow-up
OX2519	F	32	205	–	–	V179D (potentially low)	Lost to follow-up
OX312	F	38	215	–	–	K103N (high)	Lost to follow-up
OX626	F	39	550	N88S (intermediate)	–	–	Lost to follow-up

The table shows observed pre-therapy drug-associated mutations (class of antiretroviral agent, mutation position and grade of resistance), arranged in ascending order of CD4+ T-cell count and virological response (if known). [a]Grades of resistance are defined using the Stanford Drug Resistance Database. d4T, stavudine; EFV, efavirenz; F, female; M, male; VL, viral load; 3TC, lamivudine.

Table 2. Patients with drug-associated mutations to antiretroviral drugs during pre-therapy assessment

Category	PI		NRTI		NNRTI							
	M46L	N88S	T69N	K219E	A98G	K103N	V106M	V108I	E138K	179D	Y181C	Y188L
Free State Province cohort												
Patients with CD4⁺ T-cell count <100 cells/μl (n=192), n^a	1	0	2	1	2	2	1	1	1	2	2	1
Patients with CD4⁺ T-cell count 200–350 cells/μl (n=114), n^b	0	0	0	0	0	1	0	0	0	1	0	0
Patients with CD4⁺ T-cell count >500 cells/μl (n=91), n^c	0	1	0	0	0	0	0	0	0	0	0	0
Stanford drug resistance database												
Mutation prevalence in drug-naive subtype B patients, (n=7,404 for PR, n=5,539 for RT), %	0.3	0	0.4	0	0.2	0.3	0	**0.6**	0.2	**2**	0	0
Mutation prevalence in drug-naive subtype C patients (n=2,145 for PR, n=1,979 for RT), %	0.1	0	0.1	0	**0.5**	0.3	0	0.3	0.2	**0.5**	0.1	0.1
Other HIV-1 subtypes (drug-naive) with mutation prevalence ≥0.5% (subtypes A, D, F, G, AE and AG)	Subtype G (0.5%, n=619)	No	Subtype AE (0.5%, n=762)	No	No	No	No	Subtype AG (1.2%, n=1,025)	No	Subtype D (4%, n=320), subtype AE (1.5%, n=762)	No	No
Mutation prevalence in drug-experienced subtype C patients (n=282 for PR, n=1063 for RT), %	2.8	3.2	4.2	7	8.2	28	13	4	1.3	4.5	11	4.1
Genotype–treatment correlation?	Yes	Yes	Yes	Yes	Yes	Yes	Yes	Yes	Yes	Yes	Yes	Yes
Genotype–phenotype correlation?	1.8–8.2	0.1–8.9	NA	NA	NA	22–51	11–356	NA	NA	NA	1.3–148	4.3–400
Genotype–virological correlation?	Yes	Yes	Yes	Yes	Yes	Yes	Yes	NA	Yes	Yes	Yes	NA
Mutation grading (Stanford Drug Resistance Database)	Low	Intermediate	Potentially low	Low	Potentially low	High	High	Potentially low	Low	Potentially low	High	High

Table 3 shows the non-accessory drug-associated mutations in the Free State cohort and in reference cohorts (values ≥0.5% are in bold). The genotype–treatment correlation row shows whether the mutation is associated with therapy. The genotype–phenotype correlation row shows *in v tro* evidence (fold resistance) for associated phenotypic resistance. The genotype–virological correlation row shows whether mutations have an effect on viral load on therapy. All results are summarized from MARVEL and the Stanford Drug Resistance Database. The significance of each resistance mutation is compared with the drug mutation lists of the International AIDS Society-USA and the World Health Organization. *P*-values were calculated using the χ^2 test for trend, comparing the resistance statistics across the three stratified patient populations. The level of significance for clustering of mutations among low CD4⁺ T-cell counts (χ^2 test for trends) was P=0.004 for highly active antiretroviral therapy and P=0.005 for non-nucleoside reverse transcriptase inhibitors (NNRTIs). [a]Total mutations =16. [b]Total mutations =2. [c]Total mutations =1. HIV-1, HIV type-1; NA, not applicable; NRTI, nucleoside reverse transcriptase inhibitor; PI, protease inhibitor; PR, protease; RT, reverse transcriptase.

Table 3. Drug-associated mutations in the Free State Cohort

The non-accessory mutations identified in the cohort are explored in more detail in Table 3. For each mutation, the number in each CD4 T cell counts stratification is shown and compared with the reported prevalence in databases of drug-naive subtype B and C populations and in drug-experienced subtype C populations. To determine the clinical implications of these identified mutations, the Stanford database MARVEL report for each is summarized and the significance of the mutations in the surveillance lists of the WHO (updated 2009) and IAS-USA (updated December 2008) are compared (Table 3) (Bennett, et al. 2009, Johnson, et al. 2008, Stanford University 2011). For all the mutations, the prevalence in databases of drug-experienced subtype C cohorts was higher than in drug-naive patients with implications that these mutations might act as markers of drug exposure, even if not conferring clinically relevant resistance.

5.4 Enrichment of drug-associated mutations among patients with low CD4 T cell counts

Drug-associated polymorphisms (based on the Stanford database) were concentrated among patients with low CD4 T cell counts - 6.8% of patients with CD4 T cell counts <100 cells/μl carried non-accessory mutations compared with 1.8% and 1.2% of patients with intermediate and high CD4 T cell counts, respectively (P=0.015; Table 1 and Figure 4). The prevalence of resistance according to the IAS-USA definition was 3.6%, 0.9% and 1.2% for low, intermediate and high CD4 T cell counts groups, respectively (Table 1). Although not statistically significant, there were more accessory mutations among patients with low CD4 T cell counts (19.3%) compared with the intermediate (13.4%) and the high (14.0%) CD4 T cell counts groups. When using the more relaxed Stanford definition, mutations concentrated among patients with low CD4 T cell counts for all mutations (Figure 4; P=0.004). Although not statistically significant, when only considering clinically relevant mutations, there was a trend for enrichment of resistance among low CD4 T cell counts for the IAS-USA (P=0.055) and the WHO TDRM lists (P=0.086; Table 3).

In a supposedly drug-naive cohort, the enrichment of mutations with low CD4 T cell counts suggests that, rather than being transmitted, these polymorphisms had been selected by drug exposure (Garcia-Diaz, et al. 2008, Jourdain, et al. 2004). Transmitted mutations should be more common in recently infected individuals as they may revert to wild type over time in the absence of therapy (Gandhi, et al. 2003). Chronically infected patients with low CD4 T cell counts would be expected to have relatively less mutations if transmission was the only source of drug resistance. It should also be noted that other evidences have suggested that many of the transmitted resistance can stably persist over prolonged period within the HIV recipient (Brenner, et al. 2002, Novak, et al. 2005, Smith, et al. 2007). However, in the setting of this chronic cohort where majority of the patients are in advanced AIDS and HIV acquisition more likely occurred at a longer time ago, this explanation is unlikely to explain the observed drug-associated polymorphism prevalence given the availability of ARV in the distant past of SA. In this cohort, the patients were counselled by trained local HIV-1 nurses regarding drug history whether through the prevention of PMTCT, ARV programmes in different provinces, countries and private clinics or other non-governmental sources. This cohort does not comply with all the WHO guidelines for the identification of transmitted resistance (i.e. patients with recent infection, aged <25 years and no history of pregnancy (Bennett, et al. 2008, Gilks, et al. 2006, HRDS-Team 2003)), and although transmission of mutations is documented in other cohorts (Gifford, et al. 2007, Gilks, et al. 2006, Pillay 2007,

Richman, et al. 2004), a combination of phylogeny and the association with lower CD4 T cell counts in the data suggested that transmission was unlikely to be a significant cause of resistance in the Free State.

The NNRTI class, in particularly Nevirapine, was associated with significant baseline drug-associated mutations amongst the low CD4 T cell counts patient strata (Jourdain, et al. 2004). The genotypes and phylogeny of the NNRTI resistance strains were heterogenous (Figure 4 and Table 2) and were not derived from any common founder (Figure 2 and 3). Of the patients with low CD4 T cell counts (<100 cells/µl), 5.2% possessed non-nucleoside reverse transcriptase inhibitor (NNRTI)-associated mutations compared with 1.8% of patients with intermediate and 0.0% of patients with high CD4 T cell counts (P=0.005; Figure 4 and Table 3). The major mutation genotypes observed for NNRTI resistance were K103N (grade 5; 3 isolates), V106M (grade 5; 1 isolate), Y181C (grade 5; 2 isolates), and Y188L (grade 5; 1 isolate). Other NNRTI mutations included K103R (grade 1; 3 isolates), V108I (grade 2; 1 isolate), A98G (grade 2; 2 isolates), V179D (grade 2; 3 isolates), E138K (grade 3; 1 isolate), (Table 2). This association remained significant when restricted to NNRTI mutations on the IAS–USA list (P=0.031; Table 3). The distribution of NNRTI mutations within patients with

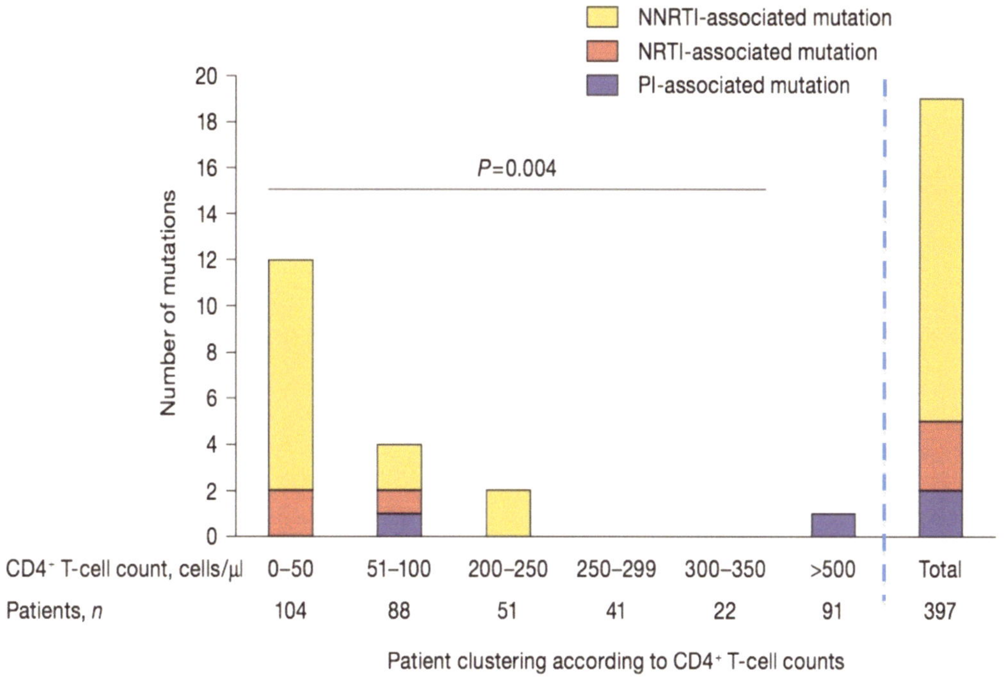

The plot depicts all pre-therapy patients carrying drug-associated mutations to any of the highly active antiretroviral therapy constituents, including protease inhibitors (PIs), nucleoside reverse transcriptase inhibitors (NRTIs) and non-nucleoside reverse transcriptase inhibitors (NNRTIs), stratified according to CD4 T cell count. The P-value was calculated using the $\chi 2$ test, comparing the mutations across CD4 T cell counts.

Fig. 4. Distribution of drug-associated mutations in pre-therapy patients according to CD4 T cell counts

low CD4 T cell counts was concentrated further among the individuals with lowest CD4 T cell counts (Table 2), who also tended to have higher grade resistant mutations.

In contrast, the prevalence of resistance to non-NNRTI classes of HAART was much lower (Table 2 and 3). Only two major PI resistance mutations in *protease* were observed (M46L (grade 3) and N88S (grade 4)) and two NRTI mutations (T69N (grade 2) and K219E (grade 3)).

Very few individuals were identified with clusters of mutations, indicative of potential multi-class resistance (Table 2). One patient (OX927) had significant resistance to both NRTI (K219E) and NNRTI (Y181C). One patient (OX1082) possessed two significant NNRTI resistance mutations, V106M and Y188L. Another (OX2032) carried E138K and Y181C.

A key route of ARV exposure is the nevirapine-only regimen initially used for PMTCT from 2000 (Department of Health 2003, Jourdain, et al. 2004, Shekelle, et al. 2007). Those patients with major NNRTI mutations were predominantly women of child-bearing age. Nevirapine is an inexpensive and effective agent and a key constituent of HAART regimens in resource-limited settings. In this cohort, nevirapine had the highest prevalence of drug-associated mutations. The drug has a long half-life, a simple mutational pathway and is prone to rapid resistance even with the single doses used in PMTCT (Grossman, et al. 2004, Jourdain, et al. 2004, Shekelle, et al. 2007). Unfortunately, despite contacting or visiting the referring clinics, the demographic details to determine the extent of this effect were not available for this analysis because of loss of follow-up for most of the affected patients.

5.5 Mathematical modelling of acquisition of drug resistance

The presence of inducible drug-resistance mutations in a population prior to recruitment to the ARV program indicates either access to antiretroviral therapy from alternative routes or transmission of drug-resistant strains. A mathematical model was developed to address two questions. Firstly, how long would it take for the observed level of inducible resistance mutation prevalence to develop in the absence of non-governmental access to drugs? Secondly, if alternative routes of drug access are maintained at the current rates, what is the likely prevalence of drug resistance in the next ten years?

Regarding the first question on the attributable impact on baseline inducible drug resistance of non-governmental access to ARVs, the model estimates that it should take between 20 and 35 years for a treatment naïve population exposed to NNRTI as part of HAART to achieve the observed level of resistance in the Free State cohort (Figure 5a). This supports the existence of additional sources of NNRTI exposure and that the Free State population is not entirely treatment naïve before the government program.

In answer to the second question, the model predicts that in patients with low CD4 T cell counts the prevalence of NNRTI resistance will increase to 7.1% (confidence interval (CI): 5.7 to 8.2%) over the next 10 years, if the additional sources of NNRTI exposure are maintained (Figure 5b). The resistance prevalence can however be stabilised to 5.2% (CI = 3.6 to 6.2%) over next 10 years, if additional exposure to NNRTI causing resistance can be reduced to 1% (currently 4.2%, Figure 5c). If all additional NNRTI exposure could be restricted, the present resistance prevalence could not sustain itself and would be expect to fall.

Therefore, according to the mathematical model, the prevalence of NNRTI resistance is likely to increase, if additional non-governmental ART exposure is not controlled. The

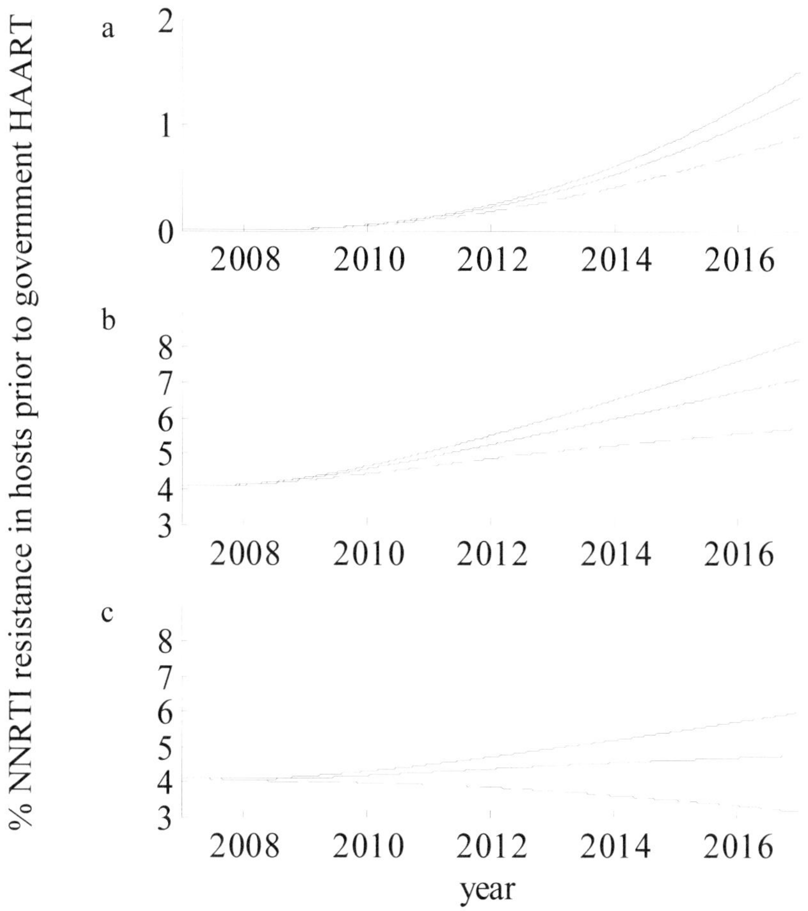

Panel A: A projection of how resistance would develop in the absence of alternative, non-governmental sources of ARTs, if there was no initial resistance to NNRTI.
Panel B: A projection of how NNRTI resistance will increase over the next 10 years if the percentage of infected hosts acquiring resistance from alternative access to therapy continues at the current level of 4% (estimated using the model).
Panel C: A projection of resistance emergence over the next 10 years, if the percentage of infected hosts acquiring resistance from alternative access to therapy reduces to 1%.
Limited data were available to estimate the rate at which drug resistant virus reverts to drug sensitive virus in untreated hosts (ψ), hence all model predictions were made for three different reversion rates: ψ = 0.13 years^{-1} (dashed line), ψ = 0.05 years^{-1} (solid line) and ψ = 0.01 years^{-1} (dotted line).

Fig. 5. Model predictions of how the prevalence of NNRTI resistance in hosts, prior to enrolment onto governmental ARTs, is expected to develop over time in the Free-State population

implications of this would include reduced drug efficacy and a requirement for clinical drug resistance surveillance, with its inherent financial costs. Newer antiretroviral classes, such as integrase and CCR5 inhibitors are currently unavailable through SA government programs re-enforcing the need to preserve the NNRTI class (Department of Health 2003). In

December 2007, South Africa revised its PMTCT regimen to a combination of zidovudine and nevirapine. Although this measure should improve PMTCT efficacy and reduce the emergence of NNRTI resistance, the logistics of introducing this change might delay its implementation in all areas of South Africa and a proportion of mothers might still receive nevirapine monotherapy.

Nonetheless, PMTCT cannot be responsible for all the observed resistance in the cohort - 6 of the 16 patients were men and the age of the females ranged from 25 to 56 years. These patients predominantly had lower grade mutations, suggestive of exposure but not clinical resistance. It is possible that some individuals had previously received treatment in other clinics, for example, contract workers travelling between provinces. In addition, patients with lower CD4 T cell counts are more likely to be symptomatic, to use drugs prescribed to family or friends and might have previously sought medication through other non-government sources (Novak, et al. 2005, Uy, et al. Jul 2007). At the time of sampling, drugs such as nevirapine, lamivudine, stavudine and didanosine were also available through private practitioners in the Free State, although the duration for which drugs would be prescribed is dependent on the patient's ability to pay (Dahab, et al. 2008, Garcia-Diaz, et al. 2008).

6. Conclusion

In summary, this chapter has reviewed the molecular epidemiology and the practical implications for HIV drug resistance testing in sub-Saharan Africa. The example study of a large cohort from South Africa has revealed new molecular epidemiological and drug resistance surveillance data. The prevalence of drug-associated mutations among patients is reassuringly low, but the association with low CD4 T cell counts is previously undescribed and warrants close monitoring of the virological response when these patients start therapy. In particular, with increasing access to antiretrovirals and growing evidence for the role of treatment as prevention, continued robust resistance surveillance mechanisms will be required for the foreseeable future.

Funding and Competing Interests: K-HGH is supported by the Rhodes Scholarships and James Martin 21st Century School. JF is funded by the Medical Research Council. The funders had no role in study design, data collection and analysis, decision to publish, or preparation of the manuscript. The data presented here have been presented at international conferences and in peer-reviewed journals prior to this publication.

Competing interests: The authors have declared that no competing interests exist.

7. References

[1] Aboulker, J. P., and A. M. Swart. 1993. Preliminary analysis of the Concorde trial. Concorde Coordinating Committee. Lancet 341:889-90.

[2] Armstrong, K. L., T. H. Lee, and M. Essex. 2009. Replicative capacity differences of thymidine analog resistance mutations in subtype B and C human immunodeficiency virus type 1. J Virol 83:4051-9.

[3] ASSA. 2007. ASSA 2003 Demographic Model Produced by the Actuarial Society of South Africa. Demographic Model. ASSA.

[4] Barbaro, G., A. Scozzafava, A. Mastrolorenzo, and C. T. Supuran. 2005. Highly active antiretroviral therapy: current state of the art, new agents and their pharmacological interactions useful for improving therapeutic outcome. Curr Pharm Des 11:1805-43.

[5] Bennett, D. E., R. J. Camacho, D. Otelea, D. R. Kuritzkes, H. Fleury, M. Kiuchi, W. Heneine, R. Kantor, M. R. Jordan, J. M. Schapiro, A. M. Vandamme, P. Sandstrom, C. A. Boucher, D. van de Vijver, S. Y. Rhee, T. F. Liu, D. Pillay, and R. W. Shafer. 2009. Drug resistance mutations for surveillance of transmitted HIV-1 drug-resistance: 2009 update. PLoS ONE 4:e4724.

[6] Bennett, D. E., M. Myatt, S. Bertagnolio, D. Sutherland, and C. F. Gilks. 2008. Recommendations for surveillance of transmitted HIV drug resistance in countries scaling up antiretroviral treatment. Antivir Ther 13 Suppl 2:25-36.

[7] Bessong, P. O., J. Mphahlele, I. A. Choge, L. C. Obi, L. Morris, M. L. Hammarskjold, and D. M. Rekosh. 2006. Resistance mutational analysis of HIV type 1 subtype C among rural South African drug-naive patients prior to large-scale availability of antiretrovirals. AIDS Res Hum Retroviruses 22:1306-12.

[8] Brenner, B. G., J. P. Routy, M. Petrella, D. Moisi, M. Oliveira, M. Detorio, B. Spira, V. Essabag, B. Conway, R. Lalonde, R. P. Sekaly, and M. A. Wainberg. 2002. Persistence and fitness of multidrug-resistant human immunodeficiency virus type 1 acquired in primary infection. J Virol 76:1753-61.

[9] Bussmann, H., V. Novitsky, W. Wester, T. Peter, K. Masupu, L. Gabaitiri, S. Kim, S. Gaseitsiwe, T. Ndungu, R. Marlink, I. Thior, and M. Essex. 2005. HIV-1 subtype C drug-resistance background among ARV-naive adults in Botswana. Antivir Chem Chemother 16:103-15.

[10] Carvajal-Rodriguez, A., K. A. Crandall, and D. Posada. 2007. Recombination favors the evolution of drug resistance in HIV-1 during antiretroviral therapy. Infect Genet Evol 7:476-83.

[11] Dahab, M., S. Charalambous, R. Hamilton, K. Fielding, K. Kielmann, G. J. Churchyard, and A. D. Grant. 2008. "That is why I stopped the ART": patients' & providers' perspectives on barriers to and enablers of HIV treatment adherence in a South African workplace programme. BMC Public Health 8:63.

[12] de Oliveira, T., and S. Cassol. 2011. The BioAfrica website, 2011 (accessible at: http://www.bioafrica.net). South African National Bioinformatics Institute.

[13] de Oliveira, T., K. Deforche, S. Cassol, M. Salminen, D. Paraskevis, C. Seebregts, J. Snoeck, E. J. van Rensburg, A. M. Wensing, D. A. van de Vijver, C. A. Boucher, R. Camacho, and A. M. Vandamme. 2005. An automated genotyping system for analysis of HIV-1 and other microbial sequences. Bioinformatics 21:3797-800.

[14] Department of Health, S. A. 2003. Operational Plan for Comprehensive HIV and Aids Care, Management and Treatment for South Africa. *In* S. A. Department of Health (ed.).

[15] DHHS-Panel. 2011. Guidelines for the use of antiretroviral agents in HIV-1-infected adults and adolescents. , p. 1–166. *In* D. o. H. a. H. Services. (ed.). Panel on Antiretroviral Guidelines for Adults and Adolescents.

[16] Egger, M., B. Hirschel, P. Francioli, P. Sudre, M. Wirz, M. Flepp, M. Rickenbach, R. Malinverni, P. Vernazza, and M. Battegay. 1997. Impact of new antiretroviral

combination therapies in HIV infected patients in Switzerland: prospective multicentre study. Swiss HIV Cohort Study. Bmj 315:1194-9.

[17] Eshleman, S. H., O. Laeyendecker, N. Parkin, W. Huang, C. Chappey, A. C. Paquet, D. Serwadda, S. J. Reynolds, N. Kiwanuka, T. C. Quinn, R. Gray, and M. Wawer. 2009. Antiretroviral drug susceptibility among drug-naive adults with recent HIV infection in Rakai, Uganda. Aids 23:845-52.

[18] Fairall, L. R., M. O. Bachmann, G. M. Louwagie, C. van Vuuren, P. Chikobvu, D. Steyn, G. H. Staniland, V. Timmerman, M. Msimanga, C. J. Seebregts, A. Boulle, R. Nhiwatiwa, E. D. Bateman, M. F. Zwarenstein, and R. D. Chapman. 2008. Effectiveness of antiretroviral treatment in a South African program: a cohort study. Arch Intern Med 168:86-93.

[19] Frater, A. J., A. Beardall, K. Ariyoshi, D. Churchill, S. Galpin, J. R. Clarke, J. N. Weber, and M. O. McClure. 2001. Impact of baseline polymorphisms in RT and protease on outcome of highly active antiretroviral therapy in HIV-1-infected African patients. Aids 15:1493-502.

[20] Frater, A. J., H. Brown, A. Oxenius, H. F. Gunthard, B. Hirschel, N. Robinson, A. J. Leslie, R. Payne, H. Crawford, A. Prendergast, C. Brander, P. Kiepiela, B. D. Walker, P. J. Goulder, A. McLean, and R. E. Phillips. 2007. Effective T-cell responses select human immunodeficiency virus mutants and slow disease progression. J Virol 81:6742-51.

[21] Frater, A. J., D. T. Dunn, A. J. Beardall, K. Ariyoshi, J. R. Clarke, M. O. McClure, and J. N. Weber. 2002. Comparative response of African HIV-1-infected individuals to highly active antiretroviral therapy. Aids 16:1139-46.

[22] Frater, J. 2002. The impact of HIV-1 subtype on the clinical response on HAART. J HIV Ther 7:92-6.

[23] Gandhi, R. T., A. Wurcel, E. S. Rosenberg, M. N. Johnston, N. Hellmann, M. Bates, M. S. Hirsch, and B. D. Walker. 2003. Progressive reversion of human immunodeficiency virus type 1 resistance mutations in vivo after transmission of a multiply drug-resistant virus. Clin Infect Dis 37:1693-8.

[24] Garcia-Diaz, A., C. Blok, S. Madge, C. Booth, M. Tyrer, S. Bonora, T. Mahungu, A. Owen, M. Johnson, and A. M. Geretti. 2008. Detection of low-frequency K103N mutants after unstructured discontinuation of efavirenz in the presence of the CYP2B6 516 TT polymorphism. J Antimicrob Chemother 62:1188-90.

[25] Garcia-Lerma, J. G., H. MacInnes, D. Bennett, H. Weinstock, and W. Heneine. 2004. Transmitted human immunodeficiency virus type 1 carrying the D67N or K219Q/E mutation evolves rapidly to zidovudine resistance in vitro and shows a high replicative fitness in the presence of zidovudine. J Virol 78:7545-52.

[26] Gifford, R. J., T. de Oliveira, A. Rambaut, O. G. Pybus, D. Dunn, A. M. Vandamme, P. Kellam, and D. Pillay. 2007. Phylogenetic surveillance of viral genetic diversity and the evolving molecular epidemiology of human immunodeficiency virus type 1. J Virol 81:13050-6.

[27] Gilks, C. F., S. Crowley, R. Ekpini, S. Gove, J. Perriens, Y. Souteyrand, D. Sutherland, M. Vitoria, T. Guerma, and K. De Cock. 2006. The WHO public-health approach to antiretroviral treatment against HIV in resource-limited settings. Lancet 368:505-10.

[28] Gordon, M., T. De Oliveira, K. Bishop, H. M. Coovadia, L. Madurai, S. Engelbrecht, E. Janse van Rensburg, A. Mosam, A. Smith, and S. Cassol. 2003. Molecular

characteristics of human immunodeficiency virus type 1 subtype C viruses from KwaZulu-Natal, South Africa: implications for vaccine and antiretroviral control strategies. J Virol 77:2587-99.
[29] Grossman, Z., V. Istomin, D. Averbuch, M. Lorber, K. Risenberg, I. Levi, M. Chowers, M. Burke, N. Bar Yaacov, and J. M. Schapiro. 2004. Genetic variation at NNRTI resistance-associated positions in patients infected with HIV-1 subtype C. Aids 18:909-15.
[30] Guindon, S., and O. Gascuel. 2003. A simple, fast, and accurate algorithm to estimate large phylogenies by maximum likelihood. Systematic Biology:8.
[31] Hamers, R. L., M. Siwale, C. L. Wallis, M. Labib, R. van Hasselt, W. S. Stevens, R. Schuurman, A. M. Wensing, M. Van Vugt, and T. F. Rinke de Wit. 2010. HIV-1 drug resistance mutations are present in six percent of persons initiating antiretroviral therapy in Lusaka, Zambia. J Acquir Immune Defic Syndr 55:95-101.
[32] HRDS-Team. 2003. Guidelines for Surveillance of HIV Drug Resistance. Guideline. WHO.
[33] Huang, K. H., D. Goedhals, H. Fryer, C. van Vuuren, A. Katzourakis, T. De Oliveira, H. Brown, S. Cassol, C. Seebregts, A. McLean, P. Klenerman, R. Phillips, and J. Frater. 2009. Prevalence of HIV type-1 drug-associated mutations in pre-therapy patients in the Free State, South Africa. Antivir Ther 14:975-84.
[34] Johnson, V. A., F. Brun-Vezinet, B. Clotet, H. F. Gunthard, D. R. Kuritzkes, D. Pillay, J. M. Schapiro, and D. D. Richman. 2008. Update of the Drug Resistance Mutations in HIV-1. Top HIV Med 16:138-45.
[35] Jourdain, G., N. Ngo-Giang-Huong, S. Le Coeur, C. Bowonwatanuwong, P. Kantipong, P. Leechanachai, S. Ariyadej, P. Leenasirimakul, S. Hammer, and M. Lallemant. 2004. Intrapartum exposure to nevirapine and subsequent maternal responses to nevirapine-based antiretroviral therapy. N Engl J Med 351:229-40.
[36] Kamoto, K., and J. Aberle-Grasse. 2008. Surveillance of transmitted HIV drug resistance with the World Health Organization threshold survey method in Lilongwe, Malawi. Antivir Ther 13 Suppl 2:83-7.
[37] Kantor, R., D. A. Katzenstein, B. Efron, A. P. Carvalho, B. Wynhoven, P. Cane, J. Clarke, S. Sirivichayakul, M. A. Soares, J. Snoeck, C. Pillay, H. Rudich, R. Rodrigues, A. Holguin, K. Ariyoshi, M. B. Bouzas, P. Cahn, W. Sugiura, V. Soriano, L. F. Brigido, Z. Grossman, L. Morris, A. M. Vandamme, A. Tanuri, P. Phanuphak, J. N. Weber, D. Pillay, P. R. Harrigan, R. Camacho, J. M. Schapiro, and R. W. Shafer. 2005. Impact of HIV-1 subtype and antiretroviral therapy on protease and reverse transcriptase genotype: results of a global collaboration. PLoS Med 2:e112.
[38] Kiepiela, P., A. J. Leslie, I. Honeyborne, D. Ramduth, C. Thobakgale, S. Chetty, P. Rathnavalu, C. Moore, K. J. Pfafferott, L. Hilton, P. Zimbwa, S. Moore, T. Allen, C. Brander, M. M. Addo, M. Altfeld, I. James, S. Mallal, M. Bunce, L. D. Barber, J. Szinger, C. Day, P. Klenerman, J. Mullins, B. Korber, H. M. Coovadia, B. D. Walker, and P. J. Goulder. 2004. Dominant influence of HLA-B in mediating the potential co-evolution of HIV and HLA. Nature 432:769-75.
[39] Kuritzkes, D. R. 2007. HIV resistance: frequency, testing, mechanisms. Top HIV Med 15:150-4.
[40] Larder, B. A., P. Kellam, and S. D. Kemp. 1993. Convergent combination therapy can select viable multidrug-resistant HIV-1 in vitro. Nature 365:451-3.

[41] Larder, B. A., S. D. Kemp, and P. R. Harrigan. 1995. Potential mechanism for sustained antiretroviral efficacy of AZT-3TC combination therapy. Science 269:696-9.
[42] Lihana, R. W., S. A. Khamadi, K. Lubano, R. Lwembe, M. K. Kiptoo, N. Lagat, J. G. Kinyua, F. A. Okoth, E. M. Songok, E. P. Makokha, and H. Ichimura. 2009. HIV type 1 subtype diversity and drug resistance among HIV type 1-infected Kenyan patients initiating antiretroviral therapy. AIDS Res Hum Retroviruses 25:1211-7.
[43] Los Alamos National Laboratory, L. 2011. HIV Databases. Los Alamos National Security, LLC.
[44] Mosha, F., W. Urassa, S. Aboud, E. Lyamuya, E. Sandstrom, H. Bredell, and C. Williamson. 2011. Prevalence of genotypic resistance to antiretroviral drugs in treatment-naive youths infected with diverse HIV type 1 subtypes and recombinant forms in Dar es Salaam, Tanzania. AIDS Res Hum Retroviruses 27:377-82.
[45] Novak, R. M., L. Chen, R. D. MacArthur, J. D. Baxter, K. Huppler Hullsiek, G. Peng, Y. Xiang, C. Henely, B. Schmetter, J. Uy, M. van den Berg-Wolf, and M. Kozal. 2005. Prevalence of antiretroviral drug resistance mutations in chronically HIV-infected, treatment-naive patients: implications for routine resistance screening before initiation of antiretroviral therapy. Clin Infect Dis 40:468-74.
[46] Palella, F. J., Jr., K. M. Delaney, A. C. Moorman, M. O. Loveless, J. Fuhrer, G. A. Satten, D. J. Aschman, and S. D. Holmberg. 1998. Declining morbidity and mortality among patients with advanced human immunodeficiency virus infection. HIV Outpatient Study Investigators. N Engl J Med 338:853-60.
[47] Pieniazek, D., M. Rayfield, D. J. Hu, J. Nkengasong, S. Z. Wiktor, R. Downing, B. Biryahwaho, T. Mastro, A. Tanuri, V. Soriano, R. Lal, and T. Dondero. 2000. Protease sequences from HIV-1 group M subtypes A-H reveal distinct amino acid mutation patterns associated with protease resistance in protease inhibitor-naive individuals worldwide. HIV Variant Working Group. Aids 14:1489-95.
[48] Pillay, C., H. Bredell, J. McIntyre, G. Gray, and L. Morris. 2002. HIV-1 subtype C reverse transcriptase sequences from drug-naive pregnant women in South Africa. AIDS Res Hum Retroviruses 18:605-10.
[49] Pillay, D. 2007. The priorities for antiviral drug resistance surveillance and research. J Antimicrob Chemother 60 Suppl 1:i57-8.
[50] Prado, J. G., T. Wrin, J. Beauchaine, L. Ruiz, C. J. Petropoulos, S. D. Frost, B. Clotet, R. T. D'Aquila, and J. Martinez-Picado. 2002. Amprenavir-resistant HIV-1 exhibits lopinavir cross-resistance and reduced replication capacity. AIDS 16:1009-17.
[51] Richman, D. D., S. C. Morton, T. Wrin, N. Hellmann, S. Berry, M. F. Shapiro, and S. A. Bozzette. 2004. The prevalence of antiretroviral drug resistance in the United States. Aids 18:1393-401.
[52] Robertson, D. L., J. P. Anderson, J. A. Bradac, J. K. Carr, B. Foley, R. K. Funkhouser, F. Gao, B. H. Hahn, M. L. Kalish, C. Kuiken, G. H. Learn, T. Leitner, F. McCutchan, S. Osmanov, M. Peeters, D. Pieniazek, M. Salminen, P. M. Sharp, S. Wolinsky, and B. Korber. 2000. HIV-1 nomenclature proposal. Science 288:55-6.
[53] Sanches, M., S. Krauchenco, N. H. Martins, A. Gustchina, A. Wlodawer, and I. Polikarpov. 2007. Structural characterization of B and non-B subtypes of HIV-protease: insights into the natural susceptibility to drug resistance development. J Mol Biol 369:1029-40.

[54] SATuRN-Database, S. Y. Rhee, T. Liu, T. de Oliveira, and R. W. Shafer. 2011. SATuRN - Southern African Treatment and Resistance Network and the Stanford HIV Drug Resistance Database (http://www.bioafrica.net/saturn/).
[55] Seebregts, C. J., C. van Vuuren, D. Goedhals, T. de Oliveira, P. Drew, P. Makhoahle, R. Nhiwatiwa, V. Timmerman, F. L., E. Kotze, R. Chapman, and S. Cassol. 5-8 June 2007. Baseline Characterization and Resistance Genotyping of HIV from the Public Sector Antiretroviral Treatment Program in the Free State Province of South Africa, The Third South African AIDS Conference, Durban, South Africa.
[56] Shafer, R. W., S. Y. Rhee, D. Pillay, V. Miller, P. Sandstrom, J. M. Schapiro, D. R. Kuritzkes, and D. Bennett. 2007. HIV-1 protease and reverse transcriptase mutations for drug resistance surveillance. Aids 21:215-23.
[57] Shekelle, P., M. Maglione, M. B. Geotz, G. Wagner, Z. Wang, L. Hilton, J. Carter, S. Chen, C. Tringle, W. Mojica, and S. Newberry. 2007. Antiretroviral (ARV) drug resistance in the developing world. Evid Rep Technol Assess (Full Rep):1-74.
[58] Smith, D. M., J. K. Wong, H. Shao, G. K. Hightower, S. H. Mai, J. M. Moreno, C. C. Ignacio, S. D. Frost, D. D. Richman, and S. J. Little. 2007. Long-term persistence of transmitted HIV drug resistance in male genital tract secretions: implications for secondary transmission. J Infect Dis 196:356-60.
[59] Sow, P. S., L. F. Otieno, E. Bissagnene, C. Kityo, R. Bennink, P. Clevenbergh, F. W. Wit, E. Waalberg, T. F. Rinke de Wit, and J. M. Lange. 2007. Implementation of an antiretroviral access program for HIV-1-infected individuals in resource-limited settings: clinical results from 4 African countries. J Acquir Immune Defic Syndr 44:262-7.
[60] Stanford University, U. 2011. HIV Drug Resistance Database (http://hivdb.stanford.edu/). Stanford University.
[61] Tshabalala, M., J. Manasa, L. S. Zijenah, S. Rusakaniko, G. Kadzirange, M. Mucheche, S. Kassaye, E. Johnston, and D. A. Katzenstein. 2011. Surveillance of transmitted antiretroviral drug resistance among HIV-1 infected women attending antenatal clinics in Chitungwiza, Zimbabwe. PLoS ONE 6:e21241.
[62] UNAIDS/WHO 2011, posting date. Report on the Global HIV/AIDS Epidemic. www.unaids.org. UNAIDS. [Online.]
[63] Uy, J., C. Armon, K. Buchacz, J. Brooks, and H. Investigators. Jul 2007. Initiation of HAART at CD4 cell counts >= 350 cells/mm3 is associated with a lower prevalence of antiretroviral resistance mutations at virologic failure, 4th IAS Conference on HIV Pathogenesis, Treatment and Prevention. Kaiser Network, Sydney, Australia.
[64] van der Ryst, E., M. Kotze, G. Joubert, M. Steyn, H. Pieters, M. van der Westhuizen, M. van Staden, and C. Venter. 1998. Correlation among total lymphocyte count, absolute CD4+ count, and CD4+ percentage in a group of HIV-1-infected South African patients. J Acquir Immune Defic Syndr Hum Retrovirol 19:238-44.
[65] Velazquez-Campoy, A., M. J. Todd, S. Vega, and E. Freire. 2001. Catalytic efficiency and vitality of HIV-1 proteases from African viral subtypes. Proc Natl Acad Sci U S A 98:6062-7.
[66] Venter, W. D. F. 2005. A critical evaluation of the South African state antiretroviral programme. The Southern African Journal of HIV Medicine.
[67] Wikimedia-Commons, R.-a. a. 2010, posting date. South Africa

(http://en.wikipedia.org/wiki/South_Africa). Multi-license with GFDL and Creative Commons CC-BY-SA-2.5 and older versions (2.0 and 1.0). [Online.]

[68] Yarchoan, R., R. W. Klecker, K. J. Weinhold, P. D. Markham, H. K. Lyerly, D. T. Durack, E. Gelmann, S. N. Lehrman, R. M. Blum, D. W. Barry, and et al. 1986. Administration of 3'-azido-3'-deoxythymidine, an inhibitor of HTLV-III/LAV replication, to patients with AIDS or AIDS-related complex. Lancet 1:575-80.